Nancy J. Smyth, PhD,
Editor

Women and Girls in the Social Environment: Behavioral Perspectives

Women and Girls in the Social Environment: Behavioral Perspectives has been co-published simultaneously as *Journal of Human Behavior in the Social Environment,* Volume 7, Numbers 3/4 2003.

Pre-publication
REVIEWS,
COMMENTARIES,
EVALUATIONS . . .

"A STIMULATING AND EX-CELLENT SOURCEBOOK for any student of human behavior, whether in school or practice. This book can also contribute to research courses. Many methodologies, including both quantitative and qualitative research, have been employed."

Esther Urdang, PhD, LICSW
Author of *Human Behavior in the Social Environment: Interweaving the Inner and Outer Worlds*

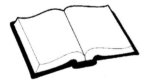

More Pre-publication
REVIEWS, COMMENTARIES, EVALUATIONS . . .

"**A**T LAST, a human behavior text in which the unit of analysis is not boys and men, but girls and women. THOROUGHLY RESEARCHED. . . . This collection would make AN EXCELLENT ADDITION TO THE STANDARD HBSE COURSE."

Katherine Van Wormer, PhD, MSSW
Professor of Social Work
University of Northern Iowa
Author of *Addiction Treatment:*
A Strengths Perspective

"**I**MPORTANT. . . . A SUPERB COLLECTION of significant studies by feminist social work scholars. . . . Offers robust new research on a broad set of critical contemporary social circumstances impinging on women in American society. The contributors exhibit superior skill in employing both illuminating qualitative analyses and sophisticated quantitative assessments. Various chapters include samples of disabled individuals, of addicted women, of lesbians, of aged grandparents raising grandchildren, and of women of color. The inclusiveness and diversity in these chapters is further enhanced by including studies of persons who span the entire life course, from girls in early childhood through women in late life."

Alan E. Bayer, PhD
Professor of Sociology
Virginia Polytechnic Institute
and State University

The Haworth Social Work Practice Press
An Imprint of The Haworth Press, Inc.

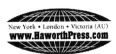

New York • London • Victoria (AU)
www.HaworthPress.com

Women and Girls
in the Social Environment:
Behavioral Perspectives

Women and Girls in the Social Environment: Behavioral Perspectives has been co-published simultaneously as *Journal of Human Behavior in the Social Environment*, Volume 7, Numbers 3/4 2003.

The *Journal of Human Behavior in the Social Environment*™ Monographic "Separates"

Below is a list of "separates," which in serials librarianship means a special issue simultaneously published as a special journal issue or double-issue *and* as a "separate" hardbound monograph. (This is a format which we also call a "DocuSerial.")

"Separates" are published because specialized libraries or professionals may wish to purchase a specific thematic issue by itself in a format which can be separately cataloged and shelved, as opposed to purchasing the journal on an on-going basis. Faculty members may also more easily consider a "separate" for classroom adoption.

"Separates" are carefully classified separately with the major book jobbers so that the journal tie-in can be noted on new book order slips to avoid duplicate purchasing.

You may wish to visit Haworth's Website at . . .

http://www.HaworthPress.com

. . . to search our online catalog for complete tables of contents of these separates and related publications.

You may also call 1-800-HAWORTH (outside US/Canada: 607-722-5857), or Fax 1-800-895-0582 (outside US/Canada: 607-771-0012), or e-mail at:

docdelivery@haworthpress.com

Women and Girls in the Social Environment: Behavioral Perspectives*,* edited by Nancy J. Smyth, PhD, CSW, CASAC (Vol. 7, No. 3/4, 2003). *"At last, a human behavior text in which the unit of analysis is not boys and men, but girls and women. Throughly researched. . . . This collection would make an excellent addition to the standard HBSE course." (Katherine van Wormer, PhD, MSSW, Professor of Social Work, University of Northern Iowa; Author of Addiction Treatment: A Strengths Perspective)*

Charting the Impacts of University-Child Welfare Collaboration*,* edited by Katharine Briar-Lawson, PhD, and Joan Levy Zlotnik, PhD, ACSW (Vol. 7, No. 1/2, 2003). *"An excellent comprehensive compilation of Title-IVE collaborations between public child welfare agencies and university settings at both BSW and MSW levels . . . " (Rowena Fong, MSW, EdD, Professor of Social Work, The University of Texas at Austin)*

Latino/Hispanic Liaisons and Visions for Human Behavior in the Social Environment*,* edited by José B. Torres, PhD, MSW, and Felix G. Rivera, PhD (Vol. 5, No. 3/4, 2002). *"An excellent example of scholarship by Latinos, for Latinos . . . . Quite useful for graduate social work courses in human behavior or social research." (Carmen Ortiz Hendricks, DSW, Associate Professsor, Hunter College School of Social Work, New York City)*

Violence as Seen Through a Prism of Color*,* edited by Letha A. (Lee) See, PhD (Vol. 4, No. 2/3, 4, 2001). *"Incisive and important. . . . A comprehensive analysis of the way violence affects people of color. Offers important insights. . . . Should be consulted by academics, students, policymakers, and members of the public." (Dr. James Midgley, Harry and Riva Specht, Professor and Dean, School of Social Welfare, University of California at Berkeley)*

Psychosocial Aspects of the Asian-American Experience: Diversity Within Diversity*,* edited by Namkee G. Choi, PhD (Vol. 3, No. 3/4, 2000). *Examines the childhood, adolescence, young adult, and aging stages of Asian Americans to help researchers and practitioners offer better services to this ethnic group. Representing Chinese, Japanese, Filipinos, Koreans, Asian Indians, Vietnamese, Hmong, Cambodians, and native-born Hawaiians, this helpful book will enable you to offer clients relevant services that are appropriate for your clients' ethnic backgrounds, beliefs, and experiences.*

Voices of First Nations People: Human Services Considerations*,* edited by Hilary N. Weaver, DSW (Vol. 2, No. 1/2, 1999). *"A must read for anyone interested in gaining an insight into the world of Native Americans. . . . I highly recommend it!" (James Knapp, BS, Executive Director, Native American Community Services of Erie and Niagara Counties, Inc., Buffalo, New York)*

Human Behavior in the Social Environment from an African American Perspective*,* edited by Letha A. (Lee) See, PhD (Vol. 1, No. 2/3, 1998). *"A book of scholarly, convincing, and relevant chapters that provide an African-American perspective on human behavior and the social environment . . . offer[s] new insights about the impact of race on psychosocial development in American society." (Alphonso W. Haynes, EdD, Professor, School of Social Work, Grand Valley State University, Grand Rapids, Michigan)*

Women and Girls
in the Social Environment:
Behavioral Perspectives

Nancy J. Smyth, PhD, CSW, CASAC
Editor

Women and Girls in the Social Environment: Behavioral Perspectives has been co-published simultaneously as *Journal of Human Behavior in the Social Environment*, Volume 7, Numbers 3/4 2003.

The Haworth Social Work Practice Press
An Imprint of
The Haworth Press, Inc.
New York • London • Oxford

Published by

The Haworth Social Work Practice Press, 10 Alice Street, Binghamton, NY 13904-1580 USA

The Haworth Social Work Practice Press is an imprint of The Haworth Press, Inc., 10 Alice Street, Binghamton, NY 13904-1580 USA.

Women and Girls in the Social Environment: Behavioral Perspectives has been co-published simultaneously as *Journal of Human Behavior in the Social Environment*, Volume 7, Numbers 3/4 2003.

The development, preparation, and publication of this work has been undertaken with great care. However, the publisher, employees, editors, and agents of The Haworth Press and all imprints of The Haworth Press, Inc., including The Haworth Medical Press® and The Pharmaceutical Products Press®, are not responsible for any errors contained herein or for consequences that may ensue from use of materials or information contained in this work. Opinions expressed by the author(s) are not necessarily those of The Haworth Press, Inc.

Cover design by Lora Wiggins.

Library of Congress Cataloging-in-Publication Data

Women and girls in the social environment: behavioral perspectives / Nancy J. Smyth editor.
    p. cm.
    "Co-published simultaneously as Journal of human behavior in the social environment, volume 7, numbers 3/4, 2003."
    Includes bibliographical references and index.
    ISBN 0-7890-2220-6 (hard: alk. paper)–ISBN 0-7890-2221-4 (soft: alk. paper)
    1. Women–Social conditions. 2. Girls–Social conditions. 3. Women–Psychology.
4. Girls–Psychology. I. Smyth, Nancy J. II. Journal of human behavior in the social environment.
  HQ1150.W643 2003
  305.42–dc22
                                            2003018088

Indexing, Abstracting & Website/Internet Coverage

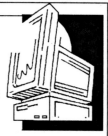

This section provides you with a list of major indexing & abstracting services. That is to say, each service began covering this periodical during the year noted in the right column. Most Websites which are listed below have indicated that they will either post, disseminate, compile, archive, cite or alert their own Website users with research-based content from this work. (This list is as current as the copyright date of this publication.)

Abstracting, Website/Indexing Coverage . . . . Year When Coverage Began

- *Cambridge Scientific Abstracts, Risk Abstracts*
  <http://www.csa.com> **1998**

- *caredata CD: the social & community care database*
  <http://www.scie.org.uk> **1998**

- *Child Development Abstracts & Bibliography*
  (in print & online) <http://www.okans.edu> **1998**

- *CINAHL (Cumulative Index to Nursing & Allied Health*
  Literature), in print, EBSCO, and SilverPlatter, Data-Star,
  and PaperChase. (Support materials include Subject Heading
  List, Database Search Guide, and instructional video)
  <http://www.cinahl.com> **1998**

- *CNPIEC Reference Guide: Chinese National Directory*
  of Foreign Periodicals **1998**

- *Criminal Justice Abstracts* **1998**

- *Environmental Sciences and Pollution Management*
  (Cambridge Scientific Abstracts Internet Database Service)
  <http://www.csa.com> . . . . *

- *e-psyche, LLC <http://www.e-psyche.net>* **2002**

- *Family & Society Studies Worldwide <http://www.nisc.com>* **1998**

- *Family Index Database <http://www.familyscholar.com>* . . . . *

(continued)

*Exact start date to come.

Special Bibliographic Notes related to special journal issues (separates) and indexing/abstracting:

- indexing/abstracting services in this list will also cover material in any "separate" that is co-published simultaneously with Haworth's special thematic journal issue or DocuSerial. Indexing/abstracting usually covers material at the article/chapter level.
- monographic co-editions are intended for either non-subscribers or libraries which intend to purchase a second copy for their circulating collections.
- monographic co-editions are reported to all jobbers/wholesalers/approval plans. The source journal is listed as the "series" to assist the prevention of duplicate purchasing in the same manner utilized for books-in-series.
- to facilitate user/access services all indexing/abstracting services are encouraged to utilize the co-indexing entry note indicated at the bottom of the first page of each article/chapter/contribution.
- this is intended to assist a library user of any reference tool (whether print, electronic, online, or CD-ROM) to locate the monographic version if the library has purchased this version but not a subscription to the source journal.

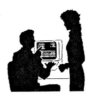

ABOUT THE EDITOR

Nancy J. Smyth, PhD, CSW, CASAC, is Associate Professor at the University at Buffalo School of Social Work, where she also chairs the MSW Concentration in Alcohol and Other Drug Problems. In addition, she is an associate research scientist at the Research Institute on Addictions in Buffalo, NY. Dr. Smyth conducts research on the problems of traumatized women, women with coexisting psychiatric and substance abuse disorders, and translating research into practice. She is Co-Principal Investigator on a grant from the National Institute on Alcohol Abuse and Alcoholism (Principal Investigator: Dr. Brenda Miller) investigating the impact of alcohol/drug problems and childhood and adulthood victimization on women's parenting. Dr. Smyth has been featured in a National Teleconference on Domestic Violence sponsored by the National Addiction Technology Transfer Center and was the lead author on the module on Women and Alcohol for the National Institute on Alcohol Abuse and Alcoholism social work curriculum.

Dr. Smyth also is Clinical Social Worker and Co-Director of the Buffalo Center for Trauma and Loss, and specializes in the treatment of survivors of psychological trauma, especially women who have been sexually abused. She has developed and consulted on treatment programs for addicted women, published on parenting issues for women with substance abuse problems, and has provided consultation to other researchers on issues related to addicted women and their parenting.

Women and Girls in the Social Environment: Behavioral Perspectives

CONTENTS

Introduction

Nancy J. Smyth

Until recently, much of our knowledge about human behavior was derived from theory or research that was based solely on men or male models of health and illness, more specifically Caucasian, middle class, men. With the advent of the second wave of feminism in the 1970s, this bias in our knowledge base was uncovered and critiqued (e.g., Gilligan, 1982; Miller, 1976). As a result, the past two decades, especially the 1990s have seen an increase in research on human behavior and practice based on women and minorities. Examination of the policies of the National Institutes of Health (NIH), the major source of federal research funding for health (including mental health and substance abuse), illustrates this trend. In the mid 1980s, in response to a Public Health Service report that identified the exclusion of women as a significant problem, the NIH established a policy encouraging the inclusion of women in federally-funded research (Pinn, Roth, Hartmuller, Bates, & Fanning, 2001). However, due to concerns about slow and uneven implementation of the policy and the lack of monitoring data, in 1994 (as a result of new legislation) the NIH began requiring that all grant applicants must address how women and minorities would be included in clinical re-

Nancy J. Smyth, PhD, CSW, CASAC, is Associate Professor, University at Buffalo School of Social Work.

Address correspondence to: Nancy J. Smyth, PhD, Associate Professor, University at Buffalo School of Social Work, 685 Baldy Hall, Buffalo, NY 14260 (E-mail: njsmyth@buffalo.edu).

[Haworth co-indexing entry note]: "Introduction." Smyth, Nancy J. Co-published simultaneously in *Journal of Human Behavior in the Social Environment* (The Haworth Social Work Practice Press, an imprint of The Haworth Press, Inc.) Vol. 7, No. 3/4, 2003, pp. 1-4; and: *Women and Girls in the Social Environment: Behavioral Perspectives* (ed: Nancy J. Smyth) The Haworth Social Work Practice Press, an imprint of The Haworth Press, Inc., 2003, pp. 1-4. Single or multiple copies of this article are available for a fee from The Haworth Document Delivery Service [1-800-HAWORTH, 9:00 a.m. - 5:00 p.m. (EST). E-mail address: docdelivery@haworthpress.com].

Digital Object Identifier: 10.1300/J137v7n03_01

search. In addition, applicants had to demonstrate that the numbers of women/minorities included in a given study were sufficient on which to base meaningful statistical analyses of gender and race effects. Although NIH research grants can still focus exclusively on one population, there must be a convincing *scientific* (not financial) rationale for doing so (Pinn et al., 2001).

In focusing on women, this special volume builds on the progress made in the last twenty years. The articles illuminate knowledge about diverse groups of women and girls, and in doing so, add significantly to our understanding of women's behavior in the context of their social environments. Given the focus of feminism on diverse ways of knowing (e.g., Belenky, Clinchy, Goldberger, & Tarule, 1986; Davis, 1987; Ivanoff, Robinson, & Blythe, 1987, 1989), it is not insignificant that the articles included here represent many ways of knowing, from the conceptual (Morrell), to the quantitative (Chapman; Dulmus, Ely, & Wodarski; Jaffee & Perloff; Robbins & Wiechelt; Williams & Lawler) and the qualitatative (Cramer, Gilson, & DePoy; Mercier & Harold; Murphy, Risley-Curtis, & Gerdes; Smyth, Miller, Mudar, & Skiba; Strother).

Some of the articles in this publication investigate important issues related to gender differences. For example, Chapman examines the use of social support by adolescent girls, compared to boys, to cope with the death of a close friend or relative, whereas Dulmus, Ely, and Wodarski compare girls' and boys' psychological responses to the victimization of a parent. While Chapman finds few gender differences, Dulmus and colleagues find that boys and girls experience very different types of psychological responses. Taken together, the articles emphasize the importance of challenging assumptions about gender differences and allowing our research to shed light on a complex phenomenon.

Several authors investigate critical topics related to childbearing and parenting. Jaffee and Perloff examine differences in ecological factors, including income and neighborhood safety, that affect health care and quality of life for White and Black mothers and their children. Exploring the resilience and strengths of mothers on welfare, Strother furthers our understanding of how these women freed themselves from poverty. Smyth, Miller, Mudar, and Skiba seek to illuminate some of the connections between addiction and victimization as they compare the ways in which mothers with and without alcohol problems protect their children. Extending the focus on parenting into an intergenerational framework, Waldrop's study of caregiving issues for grandmothers parenting their grandchildren illustrates the strain and rewards that parenting across generations creates for women. Finally, Mercier and Harold use their work with lesbian mothers to highlight an investigative tool that can communicate the richness of the relational context of women's lives.

No focus on women would be complete without articles on health. In addition to the Jaffe and Perloff article noted earlier, five articles highlight a range of women's health issues. Williams and Lawler look into social and psychological moderators of stress and illness among low-income African-American and European-American women. Extending a person-in-environment perspective further, Robbins and Wiechelt seek to illuminate connections between women's personal health behaviors and their attitudes toward caring for the environment. Given the high rates of interpersonal violence experienced by women, it is appropriate that two articles center on women's experiences with this critical social problem. Murphy, Risley-Curtiss, and Gerdes give voice to the diverse perspectives of American Indian women who have survived domestic violence, whereas Cramer, Gilson, and DePoy explore the many different types of abuse experienced by disabled women. Finally, in the last article, Morell applies empowerment theory and feminist theory to understanding women's experiences of aging and disability as they enter the *late life* phase of life.

The articles in this volume are by no means inclusive of all aspects of women's lives, nor of all women's experiences. As one reads through each contribution, the complexity and diversity around this topic becomes clear. And, as is true with all knowledge, many more questions are raised than are answered. However, each piece of work brings an important lens to our understanding of women, and each provides a perspective and focus for future work.

REFERENCES

Belenky, M.F., Clinchy, B.M., Goldberger, N.R., & Tarule, J.M. (1986). *Women's ways of knowing: The development of self, voice, and mind.* New York: Basic Books.

Davis, L.V. (1989). Empirical clinical practice from a feminist perspective: A response to Ivanoff, Robinson, and Blythe. *Social Work, 34(6),* 557-558.

Gilligan, C. (1982). *In a different voice.* Cambridge, MA: Harvard Press.

Ivanoff, A., Robinson, E.A.R., & Blythe, B. (1987). Empirical clinical practice from a feminist perspective. *Social Work, 32(5),* 417-423.

Ivanoff, A., Robinson, E.A.R., & Blythe, B. (1989). Empirical clinical practice from a feminist perspective: A response to Davis. *Social Work, 34(6),* 558-559.

Miller, J.B. (1976). *Toward a new psychology of women.* Boston: Beacon Press.

Pinn, V.W., Roth, C., Hartmuller, V.W., Bates, A., & Fanning, L. (2001, November). *Monitoring adherence to the NIH policy on the inclusion of women and minorities as subjects in clinical research: Comprehensive report (fiscal year 1998 & 1999 tracking data)* [Electronic version]. Bethesda, MD: National Institutes of Health.

Social Support and Loss During Adolescence: How Different Are Teen Girls from Boys?

Mimi V. Chapman

SUMMARY. This article describes perceived differences in social support between adolescent boys and girls who have experienced the death of a friend or relative in the last year. The article also evaluates the relative contribution of five sources of social support on adolescent girls' and boys' reports of their self-esteem, depressive symptoms, and disruptive school behavior. Boys and girls do report different levels of social support from different sources. However, the results suggest that the sources of support needed to maintain mental health and school functioning in the face of a loss are the same for boys and girls.

Mimi V. Chapman, PhD, MSW, is Assistant Professor, University of North Carolina at Chapel Hill.

Address correspondence to: Mimi V. Chapman, MSW, PhD, Assistant Professor, The University of North Carolina at Chapel Hill, School of Social Work, 301 Pittsboro Street, Campus Box 3550, Chapel Hill, NC 27599-3550 (E-mail: mimi@email.unc.edu).

The author would like to thank Drs. Gary L. Bowen and Jack M. Richman, Principal Investigators of the School Success Profile Project and Professors at the University of North Carolina at Chapel Hill School of Social Work, for the use of the data for this analysis.

[Haworth co-indexing entry note]: "Social Support and Loss During Adolescence: How Different Are Teen Girls from Boys?" Chapman, Mimi V. Co-published simultaneously in *Journal of Human Behavior in the Social Environment* (The Haworth Social Work Practice Press, an imprint of The Haworth Press, Inc.) Vol. 7, No. 3/4, 2003, pp. 5-21; and: *Women and Girls in the Social Environment: Behavioral Perspectives* (ed: Nancy J. Smyth) The Haworth Social Work Practice Press, an imprint of The Haworth Press, Inc.. 2003, pp. 5-21. Single or multiple copies of this article are available for a fee from The Haworth Document Delivery Service [1-800-HAWORTH, 9:00 a.m. - 5:00 p.m. (EST). E-mail address: docdelivery@haworthpress.com].

Digital Object Identifier: 10.1300/J137v7n03_02

KEYWORDS. Social support, loss, gender differences, adolescence

INTRODUCTION

When an adolescent experiences the death of a friend or loved one, additional social support is necessary to aid the teen in coping with the stressful life event. The increased vulnerability to depression and other potentially damaging behaviors during adolescence requires that those working with teens around a death understand which sources of support are the most valuable in helping an adolescent cope with loss (Hundley & Bratton, 1994). Previous research indicates that different sources of social support may be more important to girls versus boys, making gender differences a particularly important consideration (Colarossi & Eccles, under review). This article evaluates the relative contribution of five sources of social support on adolescent girls' and boys' reports of their self worth, depressive symptoms, and disruptive school behavior in the face of a death in the last year.

The Experience of Loss in Adolescence

Loss is not generally considered a primary area of intervention for adolescents. In fact, only recently have texts on adolescent development discussed loss and bereavement in relation to teens (Christ, 2000; Ringler & Hayden, 2000). However, the limited data available suggest that teens do experience significant deaths and that often parents and other adults have difficulty knowing how to talk with teens in the aftermath of a death (Ringler & Hayden, 2000). Certainly other points in the life course, such as old age, are more closely associated with loss and bereavement. However, the consequences of earlier grief experiences may be long lasting and significant to later functioning. Psychiatric issues, health complaints, and a host of other difficulties have been linked to grief during childhood and adolescence (Adams, Overholser, & Lehnert, 1994; Carter & Brooks, 1990; Dennehy, 1966; Raphael, 1983; Schmale & Iker, 1991). In addition, when adolescent bereavement is addressed in the literature, the focus is often on the death of parent. However, adolescents experience losses of other significant members of their social networks, including grandparents, other relatives, and peers. Peer deaths, in particular, may be considered traumatic because of their often unanticipated quality (Pynoos & Nader, 1990). Peer suicides have been associated with elevated levels of depression in teens (Brent et al., 1993). These traumatic losses may predispose teens to even more negative sequelae, particularly if caring adults are not available or knowledgeable about how to intervene.

Benefits, Sources, and Types of Social Support

Social support has been shown to be beneficial for a variety of outcomes throughout the life span (Levitt, Weber, & Guacci, 1993; Resnick, Harris, & Blum, 1993; Wyman et al., 1992). In adolescence, social support has successfully predicted levels of self-esteem, depressive symptoms, and school outcomes in teens (Barrera & Garrison-Jones, 1992; Bowen, Richman, Brewster, & Bowen, 1998; Holahan & Moos, 1987; Newcomb, 1990). School performance is positively influenced by the presence of caring others although different types of support appear to impact different school behaviors and attitudes (Rosenfeld, Richman, & Bowen, 1998). Further differentiation is seen when gender is taken into account. Although female adolescents reportedly experience closer parental and same-sex peer relationships than do males (Belle, 1989; Blythe & Foster-Clark, 1987; Noller & Callahan, 1991; Jones & Dembo, 1989), girls generally report more support from peers. Teen boys report receiving more support from family members (Berndt & Perry, 1986; Furman & Burmester, 1992; Levitt et al., 1993a). However, it is clear that the literature is mixed on the impact of gender differences in perceived support on outcomes.

To date, few authors report gender differences in social support in the face of a specific stressor event such as the death of friend or relative. However, those that do address these differences present conflicting findings—some saying that girls are more likely than boys to seek support from either peers or adults (Christ, 2000), and others describing the differential impact of peer and family support without differentiating by gender (Ringler & Hayden, 2000). This investigation seeks to enhance the current literature by examining gender differences in the types of social support needed to maintain higher levels of mental health and academic functioning in the face of a death of a peer or loved one within the last year.

METHOD

Source of Data

Data were collected between October 31, 1996 and February 15, 1997 by Louis Harris and Associates, Inc. A two-stage stratified sampling design was implemented to obtain data from a nationally representative sample of 2099 middle and high school students. A sample of 93 public middle and high schools in the United States was chosen, including 39 middle schools (6th through 8th grades) and 54 high schools (9th through 12th grades). Then a representative sample of students from the schools was selected. The sampling design was tailored to ensure adequate representation of students by gender, race/ethnicity, urbanicity of location, and region. Data were collected using the School Success Profile (SSP), a self-administered survey instrument (Richman & Bowen, 1997). This instrument was designed for Communities In Schools (CIS), the largest stay in school network in the United States. The SSP is informed by an ecological perspective and as such provides information on student perceptions of their four primary environments, school, family, friends, and neighborhoods. This self-report strategy is supported by a variety of scholars who argue that older children and teens are the best informants about their own behavior and life circumstances (Garbarino, Stott, & Faculty of the Erikson Institute, 1989; Paulson, 1996; Rosenfeld, Richman, & Bowen, 1998).

Sample

Of the 2099 students who responded to the Harris Survey, 469 students reported experiencing the death of a friend, parent, or close relative in the last year. These 469 students made up the sample used for this analysis. Females made up 58% of the sample. The majority of the sample identified themselves as White (58%), while 17% identified as African-American, 9% were Hispanic, and 15% identified as either Native American, Asian-Pacific Islander, multiracial, or as a member of some other racial/ethnic group. Eleven-through-seventeen-year-olds made up 94% of the sample. Slightly over one-quarter of the sample (28%) received a free or reduced price lunch in school. Most members of the sample lived with two parents or adults in their home (70%). Twenty percent lived in single parent families, and 10% lived in some other sort of situation.

Measures

Eight measures, including five independent variables and three outcome variables, were used to examine the relationship between five sources of social support and self worth, depressed mood, and disruptive behavior in school. In addition, five demographic variables were entered into the regression equations. Table 1 presents descriptive data on the measures used in the analysis. The correlation matrix shown in Table 2 shows a pattern of modest correlations demonstrating the relative independence of the constructs used in this analysis.

Independent Variables

Five sources of social support were assessed. *Peer Support* measured perceptions of student satisfaction with support received from same age friends. "True" responses to statements such as "I am satisfied with the way my friends respond to my feelings," were tallied and re-coded to

TABLE 1. Descriptive Information on Measures (N = 469)

Measure Name	Range	Mean	Standard Deviation	Cronbach's Alpha
Gender (1 = female)	1-2	1.42	.49	N/A
Race/Ethnicity (1 = non-white)	1-2	1.6	.49	N/A
Family Constellation (1 = single parent)	1-2	1.7	.46	N/A
Free Lunch (1 = no)	1-2	1.4	.49	N/A
Peer Support*	5-10	9.0	1.48	.80
Parent Support*	20-60	48.2	11.18	.96
Neighborhood Support*	7-14	11.2	1.80	.64
Teacher Support*	9-18	15.6	2.55	.86
General Social Support*	8-16	15.7	2.42	.77
Depressed Mood**	4-8	8.9	2.80	.79
Poor Self Worth**	5-15	6.3	2.40	.83
Disruptive Behavior**	4-8	4.7	1.00	.56

Note: N/A = not applicable.
*Higher scores indicate higher support.
**Higher scores indicate problem symptoms/behavior.

TABLE 2. Correlation Matrix–Measures in the Analysis ($\underline{N}$ = 469)

Measure Name	1.	2.	3.	4.	5.	6.	7.	8.	9.	10.	11.	12.
1. Gender	1	.06	.03	-.02	-.13	-.12	-.18	.05	.01	-.30	-.05	.10
2. Race/Ethnicity	--	1	.14	-.35	.08	-.01	-.05	.12	-.06	-.03	.05	-.10
3. Family Constellation	--	--	1	-.15	.13	.11	.15	.17	.11	-.07	-.09	-.12
4. Free Lunch	--	--	--	1	-.09	.04	.00	-.09	.00	.08	-.01	.05
5. Peer Support	--	--	--	--	1	.30	.32	.27	.24	-.11	-.21	-.16
6. Teacher Support	--	--	--	--	--	1	.31	.25	.35	-.12	-.25	-.32
7. General Social Support	--	--	--	--	--	--	1	.28	.52	-.08	-.37	-.24
8. Neighborhood Support	--	--	--	--	--	--	--	1	.32	-.25	-.27	-.16
9. Parent Support	--	--	--	--	--	--	--	--	1	-.23	-.37	-.18
10. Depressed Mood	--	--	--	--	--	--	--	--	--	1	.44	.17
11. Poor Self Worth	--	--	--	--	--	--	--	--	--	--	1	.29
12. Disruptive Behavior	--	--	--	--	--	--	--	--	--	--	--	1

create a scale ranging from 5 to 10 with higher scores indicating higher levels of peer support.

Teacher Support measured student perceptions of feelings related to teachers at their school. Summed "true" responses to statements such as "I receive a lot of encouragement from my teachers," were re-coded to create a scale ranging from 9 to 18 with higher scores indicating higher levels of teacher support.

Neighborhood Support measured the level of cohesion, encouragement, and support students perceive from their neighbors. The development of these items was informed by Small and Kerns' (1993) neighborhood monitoring scale. "Agree" responses to statements such as "People in my neighborhood really help one another out," were summed and re-coded to create scores ranging from 7 to 14 with higher scores indicating higher neighborhood support.

Parent Support assessed 20 specific supportive behaviors such as "helped you solve a problem," "gave you encouragement," "spent free time with you." A three-point response continuum was provided including never, sometimes, and often. Often responses were summed creating a scale ranging from 20 to 60 with higher scores indicating higher parental support.

Finally, *General Social Support* assessed support that could be received from anyone in the student's life. "Yes" responses were summed to create scores ranging from 8 to 16 with higher scores indicating higher levels of general social support. Alpha coefficients for the independent variables, presented in Table 1, range from .64 to .96 indicating a high level of internal consistency within each measure.

Dependent Variables

Disruptive School Behavior was assessed with four indicators of the frequency of problem behaviors in the past 30 days. Students were asked how often they had been sent out of the class due to misbehavior; whether their parents/guardians had received a warning about attendance, grades, or behavior; how often they had been helpful to others in the school setting; and if they had been suspended or expelled. These questions were adapted from NELS (National Opinion Research Center, 1988). Students could answer 1, more than twice; 2, once or twice, or 3, never. Following re-coding, summed responses ranged from 4 to 8 with higher numbers representing worse behavior.

Depressed Mood consisted of five summed items which asked students how often they experienced feelings of loneliness, fear, confusion, sadness, or wanting to cry. Responses ranged from never (1) to often (3) with scores ranging from 5 to 15 with a higher score indicating the presence of more depressive symptoms.

Self Worth was measured using a four-item scale adapted from Rosenberg's (1965) self-esteem scale. Students were asked whether statements indicating feelings of failure, not having much to be proud of, feeling no good, and feeling useless were 1, "a lot like me," 2, "a little like me," or 3, "not like me." Responses were re-coded and summed to create scores ranging from 4 to 12 with higher scores indicating poorer self worth. Alpha coefficients for the dependent variables range from .56 to .83 indicating an acceptable level of internal consistency within the constructs.

In addition, four single-item variables were included as covariates in the analysis: gender, racial/ethnic group identification, family constellation, and free or reduced price lunch. Free lunch status has been used as a proxy measure for lower socioeconomic status in previous investigations (Bowen & Chapman, 1996; Bowen & Bowen, 1999). Each of these measures was coded into dichotomous categories as noted in Table 1.

Analysis

The data were analyzed in two stages. Following examination of the correlation matrix presented in Table 2, t-tests were performed to examine difference in levels of social support by gender. A .05 level of significance was used to evaluate results from this analysis.

Next, a series of blockwise hierarchical multiple regressions was performed (Cohen & Cohen, 1975). These analyses compared the relative contribution of three sets of variables–demographics, types of social support, and gender interaction terms–in explaining variation in the three dependent variables. In addition, the full model examined the relative contributions when all variables were entered simultaneously. The approach of entering related variables in blocks allows greater potential understanding of the unique contributions of each type of variable than a simultaneous entry approach (Greenberger, Goldberg, Hamill, O'Neil, & Payne, 1989).

RESULTS

Table 3 shows the statistically significant results that emerged when the measures of social support were analyzed by gender. As hypothesized, adolescent boys and girls do perceive differences in the mean level of social support they receive. Females report higher mean levels of general social support (M = 16.09), peer support (M = 9.18), and teacher support (M = 15.81). Boys report slightly higher levels of neighborhood and parent support although these levels do not reach statistical significance. When considered within the theoretical range of each measure, both boys and girls reported moderate levels of each type of perceived support.

Hierarchical multiple regressions of the three outcome variables, self worth, depressed mood, and trouble avoidance at school on the five types of support, constituted the second level of analysis. Tables 4, 5, and 6 provide the analysis results.

Regression Results: Depressed Mood

Table 4 provides regression statistics describing the predictive value of the five types of social support for depressive symptoms. The four demographic variables explained a significant portion of the variance in depressive symptoms. Together, these variables accounted for approximately 10% of the total variance in depressive symptoms, *R square = .097, F (4, 438) = 11.71, P < .01.*

In Step 2, the five social support measures explained a significant portion of the variance beyond the contribution of the demographic variables in Step 1, *R square change = .08, F (9, 433) = 10.44, P < .01.* These five variables added approximately 8% to the variation in the

TABLE 3. Means and Standard Deviations of Measures of Social Support by Gender (N = 469)

| Support Variable | Female N = 272 | | Male N = 197 | | |
	M	SD	M	SD	t-test
Neighborhood	11.15	1.75	11.34	1.90	−1.12
Teacher	15.81	2.44	15.18	2.68	2.56**
Parent	48.10	11.61	48.22	10.59	−.117
Peer	9.18	1.37	8.80	1.59	2.72**
General	16.10	2.24	15.24	2.60	3.74***

*p < .05
**p < .01
***p < .000

TABLE 4. Hierarchical Regression–Depressed Mood (N = 469)

| Variable | Step 1 | | Step 2 | |
	B	Beta	B	Beta
Demographics				
Gender	−1.68	−.296***	−1.701	−.300***
Race/ethnicity	3.347E-02	.006	6.636E-02	.012
Family constellation	−.335	−.005	−4.364E-02	−.007
School lunch	.354	.063	.335	.059
Support				
Neighborhood			−.222	−.142**
Teacher			−6.098E-02	−.056
Parent			−4.069E-02	−.164**
Peer			−.107	−.057
General			2.393E-02	.021
Constant	11.344		16.861	
Multiple R	.311		.422	
R^2	.097		.178	
F	11.71		10.443	
$R^{2\ change}$			.082	
F			8.613	

*p < .05

**p < .01

***p < .000

TABLE 5. Hierarchical Regression–Self Worth (N = 469)

Variable	Step 1 B	Step 1 Beta	Step 2 B	Step 2 Beta
Demographics				
Gender	−.238	−.048	−.481	−.098*
Race/ethnicity	.244	.050	.194	.039
Family constellation	−.487	−.093	−4.545E-02	−.009
School lunch	−.9750E-02	−.020	−7.677E-02	−.016
Support				
Neighborhood			−.154	−.114**
Teacher			−7.280E-02	−.077
Parent			−4.053E-02	−.188***
Peer			−8.261E-02	−.051
General			−.223	−.221***
Constant	7.219		15.958	
Multiple R	.110		.470	
R^2	.012		.221	
F	1.353		13.646***	
R^2 change			.21	
F			23.206***	

*p < .05
**p < .01
***p < .000

level of depressive symptoms. When cross-product terms were entered into the model to examine the interaction between gender and the five types of social support, no significant interactions emerged. Taken together these findings indicate that social support and demographic variables have an impact on the outcome of depressive symptoms. In Step 2, gender, parent support, and neighborhood support produced statistically significant weights. The lack of significant interactions indicates that depressive symptoms in adolescents are reduced by the presence of these types of social support regardless of gender.

Regression Results: Self Worth

Table 5 contains the regression statistics describing the impact of the five types of support on self worth. In this analysis, the four demographic variables failed to explain a significant portion of the variance in self worth. Together, these variables accounted for less than 1.5% of the total variance in self worth, *R square = .01, F (4, 438) = 1.35, P > .05.*

TABLE 6. Hierarchical Regression–Disruptive School Behavior ($\underline{N}$ = 469)

Variable	Step 1 B	Step 1 Beta	Step 2 B	Step 2 Beta
Demographics				
Gender	.19	.096*	8.569E-02	.043
Race/ethnicity	−.230	−.116*	−.225	−.113*
Family constellation	−.221	−.104*	−.104	−.049
School lunch	3.197E-02	.016	7.039E-02	.035
Support				
Neighborhood			−1.222E-02	−.022
Teacher			−9.899E-02	−.260***
Parent			−3.436E-03	.040
Peer			−6.837E-03	−.010
General			−5.087E-02	−.125*
Constant	5.119		7.716	
Multiple R	.193		.396	
R^2	.037		.157	
F	4.227**		8.910***	
R^2 change			.119**	
F			12.222***	

*p < .05
**p < .01
***p < .000

However, the five social support measures added in Step 2 explained a significant portion of the variance beyond the contribution of the demographic variables in Step 1, *R square change = .21, F (9, 433)= 13.64, P < .01*. These five variables added approximately 21% to the variation in the reported self worth of students facing a loss. Again, cross-product terms were added to the model to examine potential gender interactions; however, no interactions were present. These findings indicate that social support has a greater impact than demographic variables on reported self worth. In this analysis, parent support, neighborhood support, and general social support produced significant weights. The lack of gender interactions would suggest that adolescents benefit equally from these types of support regardless of gender.

Regression Results: Disruptive School Behavior

Table 6 provides the regression statistics for depressed mood. In this analysis, the four demographic variables explained a small but significant portion of the variance in depressive symptoms. Together, these variables accounted for about 4% of the total variance in depressive symptoms, *R square = .037, F (4, 437) = 4.227, P < .01.*

Again, the five social support variables explained a significant portion of the variance beyond the contribution of the demographic variables in Step 1, *R square change = .119, F (9, 432) = 8.91, P < .000.* These five variables added approximately 12% to the variation in disruptive behavior. Cross-product terms entered into the model again revealed no interactions between gender and the five types of social support. Race/ethnicity, general social support, and teacher support produced significant weights in model 2. The types of social support needed to impact disruptive behavior do not appear to differ by gender.

DISCUSSION

The findings presented reinforce the importance of social support for adolescents in the face of a significant life stressor–in this case the death of a friend or relative. The findings do not support the idea that adolescent boys and girls benefit from different types of social support. Teen boys and girls report different levels of each of the types of support considered in this investigation. However, these differences do not seem to relate to the particular outcomes considered here. Rather, predictors of depressive symptoms, self worth, and disruptive school behavior appear to apply equally to both genders. In this analysis, girls reported receiving higher levels of teacher support, peer support, and general social support. Possible interpretations of these findings include a measurement effect related to the types of activities that are considered supportive by males and females. The types of social support girls appear to receive and want focus largely on talking, sharing emotions, and receiving affirmation. In this analysis, the parental support and neighborhood support measures contain both items that focus both on emotional types of support and more instrumental support. Clearly, young males benefit from being able to talk about their feelings; however, they may perceive support from activities and interactions that researchers have not yet captured in social support measures (Wood & Inman, 1993).

An intriguing finding involves the role of neighborhood support. Both depressive symptoms and self worth were influenced by this variable. Although it is difficult to assess the role of the larger social environment, these findings suggest that research into the impact of social context is important to understanding a variety of adolescent outcomes, particularly in light of a stressor event. A growing body of literature supports the notion that neighborhood characteristics have substantial influence on many child and adolescent outcomes (Bowen & Chapman, 1996; Brook et al., 1989; Chapman, 1997; Gonzales, Cauce, Friedman, & Mason, 1996; Klebanov, Brooks-Gunn, & Duncan, 1994; Peeples & Loeber, 1994). These findings add to that literature. At a time of great emotional upheaval, the presence and awareness of supportive neighbors who take an interest in youth may do much to buffer and reassure grieving teens.

Perhaps the most significant finding concerns the places from which teens receive social support. Depressive symptoms were most affected by levels of parent and neighborhood support. Self worth was most affected by levels of parent, neighborhood, and general social support. Finally, predictors of disruptive school behavior were limited to teacher support and general social support. What is noticeably missing in each of these analyses is the role of peer support. At least, when facing the stressor of loss, it appears to be adults, not peers, who make the difference in the lives of adolescents. This finding runs contrary to prevailing attitudes about the importance of peers in the adolescent years. Teens appear to have convinced many adults that they prefer to receive support from their peers. Yet, these findings point to a different conclusion. That is, that while teens might actively attempt to push adults out their lives, adults would do well to remain fully connected and engaged particularly when difficult life events, like a significant death, come along.

Practice Implications

For those working with grieving teens, these findings should serve to remind clinicians that both genders require extensive social support in order to maintain adequate functioning in the face of loss. These findings suggest that support comes from similar places for both teen girls and boys. Our assumptions about how gender influences a teenager's need for support may come from our own biases and stereotypes about how males and females process stressful life experiences.

In addition, these findings should remind clinicians of the powerful role of adults in adolescents' lives. Therefore, including parents, teachers, and other caring adults in the assessment and treatment planning for teens experiencing a stressor is something that should not be forgotten. Including these adults may take additional time or mean changing agency payment structures, but to ignore these "natural helpers" is to do teens a disservice.

Finally, as medical models and biological explanations for behavior become evermore present, it is tempting to ignore the broader contexts that may interact with biology to impact well-being. These findings should encourage mental health professionals to maintain a focus on the wider social environment, in this case neighborhood, to acknowledge and incorporate into interventions its potential influence in either pre-disposing or protecting and adolescent girl or boy to or from negative consequences in the face of a stressor.

Directions for Future Research

Although this analysis did not show significant differences between adolescent females and males regarding social support in the face of loss, further research into this area could provide useful information about gender differences. Qualitative inquiries concerning gender differences in social support use may be helpful in clarifying how social support is used and in creating measures that more accurately reflect behaviors that both genders consider supportive. Longitudinal explorations would allow investigators to examine the impact of different types of social support at a given point in time on outcomes further down the road. The ability to make causal linkages is limited by the cross-sectional nature of the current analysis.

CONCLUSION

When considering the impact of the social environment on human behavior, it is important to evaluate gender differences as part of any investigation. Current popular culture reinforces notions of gender differences saying "Men are from Mars; Women are from Venus," or that we live in a girl or boy hating culture (depending on the author). Certainly, gender differences cannot be denied both by virtue of socialization and biology. However, it is incumbent on social scientists to consider and evaluate these supposed differences both because of what we may learn about how boys and girls are different and because we may learn how boys and girls are the same. Stereotypes and cultural messages will forever be a part of the social environment. Thorough inquiry is required to understand what sorts of influences truly shape behavior.

REFERENCES

Adams, D.M., Overholser, J.C., & Lehnert, K.L. (1994). Perceived family functioning and adolescent suicidal behavior. *Journal of the American Academy of Child and Adolescent Psychiatry, 33*, 498-507.

Barrera, M., & Garrison-Jones, C. (1992). Family and peer social support as specific correlates of adolescent depressive symptoms. *Journal of Abnormal Child Psychology, 20*, 1-16.

Belle, D. (1989). Gender differences in children's social networks and supports. In D. Belle (Ed.), *Children's social networks and social supports* (pp. 173-188). New York: John Wiley.

Berndt, T.J., & Perry, T.B. (1986). Children's perceptions of friendships as supportive relationships. *Developmental Psychology, 22* (5), 640-648.

Blythe, D.A., & Foster-Clark, F.S. (1987). Gender differences in perceived intimacy with different members of adolescent's social networks. *Sex Roles, 17*, 689-728.

Bowen, N.K., & Bowen, G.L. (1999). Effects of crime and violence in neighborhoods and schools on the school behavior and performances of adolescents. *Journal of Adolescent Research, 14* (3), 319-342.

Bowen, G.L., & Chapman, M.V. (1996). Poverty, neighborhood danger, social support, and the individual adaptation among at-risk youth in urban areas. *Journal of Family Issues, 17* (5), 641-666.

Bowen, G.L., Richman, J.M., Brewster, A., & Bowen, N. (1998). Sense of school coherence, perceptions of danger at school, and teacher support among youth at risk of school failure. *Child and Adolescent Social Work Journal, 15 (4), 273-286.*

Brent, D.A., Perper, J.A., Moritz, G., Allman, C., Schweers, J., Roths, C., Balach, L., Canobbio, R., & Liotus, L. (1993). Psychiatric sequelae to the loss of an adolescent peer to suicide. *Journal of the American Academy of Child and Adolescent Psychiatry, 32* (3) 509-517.

Brook, J.S., Nomura, C., & Cohen, P. (1989). A network of influences on adolescent drug involvement: Neighborhood, school, peer, and family. *Genetic, Social, and General Psychology Monographs, 115* (1), 123-145.

Carter, B.F., & Brooks, A. (1990). Child and adolescent survivors of suicide. In A.A. Leenaars (Ed.), *Life span perspectives of suicide* (pp. 231-258). New York: Plenum.

Chapman, M.V. (1997). Neighborhood quality and somatic complaints among American youth. Unpublished doctoral dissertation, The University of North Carolina at Chapel Hill, Chapel Hill.

Christ, G. H. (2000). *Healing children's grief: Surviving a parent's death from cancer.* New York: Oxford Press.

Cohen, J., & Cohen, P. (1975). *Applied multiple regression/correlation analysis for the behavioral sciences.* Hillsdale, NJ: Lawrence Erlbaum.

Colarossi, L.G., & Eccles, J. S. (1999). A prospective study of adolescent peer support: Gender differences and the influence of parental relationships (unpublished manuscript).

Dennehy, C.M. (1966). Childhood bereavement and psychiatric illness. *British Journal of Psychiatry, 112,* 1049-1069.

Furman, W., & Buhrmester, D. (1992). Age and sex differences in perceptions of networks of personal relationships. *Child Development, 63,* 103-115.

Garbarino, J., Stott, F.M., & Faculty of the Erikson Institute. (1989). *What children can tell us: Eliciting, interpreting, and evaluating information from children.* San Fransisco: Jossey-Bass.

Gonzales, N., Cauce, A.M., Friedman, R.J., & Mason, C. (1996). Family, peer, and neighbhorhood influences on academic achievement among African-American adolescents: One year prospective effects. *American Journal of Community Psychology, 24* (3), 365-387.

Greenberger, E., Goldber, W.A., Hamill, S., O'Neil, R., & Payne, C.K. (1989). Contributions of a supportive work environment to parent's well-being and orientation to work. *American Journal of Community Psychology, 17,* 755-783.

Holahan, C.J., & Moos, R.H. (1987). Risk, resiliance, and psychological distress: A longitudinal analysis with adults and children. *Journal of Abnormal Psychology, 96,* 3-13.

Hundley, M., & Bratton, S. (1994). Adolescent loss and the school community: Don't let them slip through your fingers. *TCA-Journal, 22,* 10-22.

Jones, G.P., & Dembo, M.H. (1989). Age and sex role differences in intimate friendships during childhood and adolescence. *Merrill-Palmer Quarterly, 35* (4), 445-462.

Klebanov, P.K., Brooks-Gunn, J., & Duncan, G.J. (1994). Does neighborhood and family poverty affect mother's parenting, mental health, and social support. *Journal of Marriage and the Family, 56* (2), 441-455.

Levitt, M.J., Gaucci-Franco, N., & Levitt, J.L. (1993a). Convoys of social support in childhood and early adolescence: Structure and function. *Developmental Psychology, 29* (5), 811-818.

Levitt, M.J., Weber, R.A., & Gaucci, N. (1993). Convoys of social support: An intergenerational analysis. *Psychology & Aging, 8* (3), 323-326.

National Opinion Research Center. (1988). National educational longitudinal study of 1988: First follow-up questionnaire (OMB No. 1850-0593). Washington, D.C.: U.S. Department of Education, National Center for Education Statistics.

Newcomb, M.D. (1990). Social support and person characteristics: A developmental and interactional perspective. *Journal of Social and Clinical Psychology, 9* (1), 54-68.

Noller, P., & Callahan, C. (1991). *The adolescent in the family.* London: Routledge.

Paulson, S.E. (1996). Maternal employment and adolescent achievement revisited: An ecological perspective. *Family Relations, 45,* 201-208.

Peeples, F., & Loeber, R. (1994). Do individual factors and neighborhood context explain ethnic differences in juvenile delinquency? *Journal of Quantitative Criminology, 10* (2), 141-157.

Pynoos, R.S., & Nader, K. (1990). Children's exposure to violence and traumatic death. *Psychiatric Annals, 20,* 334-344.

Raphael, B. (1983). *The anatomy of bereavement.* New York: Basic Books.

Resnick, M.D., Harris, L.J., & Blum, R.W. (1993). The impact of caring and connectedness on adolescent health and well-being. *Journal of Paediatric Child Health, 29,* (Suppl.1), S3-S9.

Richman, J.M., & Bowen, G.L. (1997). School failure: An ecological-interactional-developmental perspective. In M.W. Fraser (Ed.), *Risk and resilience in childhood: An ecological perspective* (pp. 95-116). Washington, DC: NASW Press.

Ringler, L.L., & Hayden, D.C. (2000). Adolescent bereavement and social support: Peer loss compared to other losses. *Journal of Adolescent Research, 15,* 209-230.

Rosenberg, M. (1965). *Society and the adolescent self-image.* Princeton, New Jersey: Princeton University Press.

Rosenfeld, L.B., Richman, J.M., & Bowen, G.L. (1998). Low social support among at-risk adolescents. *Social Work in Education, 20,* 245-260.

Schmale, A.H., & Iker, H. (1991). Hopelessness as a predictor of cervical carcinoma. *Social Science and Medicine, 5,* 95-100.

Small, S.A., & Kerns, D. (1993). Unwanted sexual activity during early and middle adolescence: Incidence and risk factors. *Journal of Marriage and the Family, 55,* 941-952.

Wood, J.T., & Inman, C.C. (1993). In a different mode: Masculine styles of communicating closeness. *Journal of Applied Communication Research, 21,* 279-295.

Wyman, P.A., Cowen, E.L., Work, W.C., Raoof, A., Gribble, P.A., Parker, G.R., & Wannon, M. (1992). Interviews with children who experienced major life stress: Family and child attributes that predict resilient outcomes. *Journal of the American Academy of Child and Adolescent Psychiatry, 31*(5), 904-910.

Children's Psychological Response to Parental Victimization: How Do Girls and Boys Differ?

Catherine N. Dulmus
Gretchen Ely
John S. Wodarski

SUMMARY. This study found that African American children, 6 through 12 years of age, whose parents had been victims of community violence (i.e., gunshot or stabbing) experienced distress symptoms differently, depending on their gender. In the authors' previous work (Dulmus & Wodarski, 2000), children, age 6-12, whose parents were victims of community violence (e.g., gunshot, stabbing), and whose victimization the children did not witness, were found to be experiencing distress symptoms related to their parents' victimization. The purpose of

Catherine N. Dulmus, PhD, ACSW, is Assistant Professor, The University of Tennessee, College of Social Work, 301 Henson Hall, Knoxville, TN 37849 (E-mail: cdulmus@utk.edu).

Gretchen Ely, MSW, is a Doctoral Candidate, The University of Tennessee, College of Social Work, 125 Henson Hall, Knoxville, TN 37849 (E-mail: geely@utk.edu).

John S. Wodarski, PhD, is Professor and Director of Research, The University of Tennessee, College of Social Work, 822 Beale Street, Room 220, Memphis, TN 38163 (E-mail: jwodarsk@utk.edu).

The authors would like to thank the Trauma Center at Erie County Medical Center, Buffalo, NY for facilitating data collection for this project.

[Haworth co-indexing entry note]: "Children's Psychological Response to Parental Victimization: How Do Girls and Boys Differ?" Dulmus, Catherine N., Gretchen Ely, and John S. Wodarski. Co-published simultaneously in *Journal of Human Behavior in the Social Environment* (The Haworth Social Work Practice Press, an imprint of The Haworth Press, Inc.) Vol. 7, No. 3/4, 2003, pp. 23-36; and: *Women and Girls in the Social Environment: Behavioral Perspectives* (ed: Nancy J. Smyth) The Haworth Social Work Practice Press, an imprint of The Haworth Press, Inc., 2003, pp. 23-36. Single or multiple copies of this article are available for a fee from The Haworth Document Delivery Service [1-800-HAWORTH, 9:00 a.m. - 5:00 p.m. (EST). E-mail address: docdelivery@haworthpress.com].

Digital Object Identifier: 10.1300/J137v7n03_03

this current study was to do further analysis to examine children's psychological response to parental victimization by gender. Results indicated that all children in the study were experiencing symptoms in the borderline clinical range as measured by the total score on the Child Behavior Checklist (CBCL), with females having a mean score of 39.5 and males having a mean score of 38. The differences that were found by gender were in children's expression of symptoms; with females experiencing more internalizing symptoms (i.e., withdrawn, somatic complaints, anxiety, depression) and males experiencing more externalizing symptoms (i.e., aggression, delinquent behaviors). Such results support feminist theory, which suggests that girls and boys respond differently to stimuli because of gender differences related to socialization. Such distinctions may be clinically useful when choosing approaches to behavioral interventions. *[Article copies available for a fee from The Haworth Document Delivery Service: 1-800-HAWORTH. E-mail address: <docdelivery@haworthpress.com> Website: <http://www. Haworth Press.com>* © *2003 by The Haworth Press, Inc. All rights reserved.]*

KEYWORDS. Childhood trauma, gender differences, parental victimization, community violence

The United States currently has the distinction of being the most violent country in the industrialized world (Fingerhut & Kleinman, 1990). Unfortunately, this "distinction" may have grave consequences for the many American children whose daily lives include exposure to chronic community violence. Each day in the United States nine children are murdered and 30 children are wounded with guns (Children's Defense Fund, 1993). Manning and Baruth (1995) reported that approximately 28,200 students are physically attacked in American schools each month. On an average day in the United States, 65 people die from, and more than 6000 people are physically injured by, interpersonal violence (Harlow, 1989). It is estimated that approximately two million assaults occur annually in the United States, assaults that are violent enough to require a hospital emergency room visit (Barancik, 1983). Acts of violence that do not necessitate an emergency room visit are unknown.

Though crime rates have been falling for the past six years (*The Economist*, 1998), violence continues to be a public health problem in the United States. Community violence should not be discounted as a result of falling crime rates, as many urban children continue to be involved both as victims of, and eyewitnesses to, episodes of violence in their communities and schools (Richters, 1993). Some of these children have described their experiences as "living in a battle zone" (Lorion & Saltzman, 1990).

Researchers have begun to study children's exposure to chronic community violence. Chronic community violence (CCV) is defined as frequent and continual exposure in the community to the use of guns, knives, drugs, and random violence (Osofsky, 1995). Richters and Martinez (1993) examined exposure to CCV of children living in a low-income, moderately violent neighborhood in Washington, DC; of these, 61% reported that they had witnessed violence to someone else, and 19% reported that they themselves had been victimized. Osofsky, Wewers, Hann, and Fick (1993) further documented that 26% of mothers in a New Orleans housing project had seen shootings, while 49% of their children had seen others become wounded, and more than 70% of their children had seen weapons used. What are the consequences to the mental health of these children who are chronically exposed to community violence?

Unfortunately, there has been little systematic research to date concerning the psychological consequences to children being raised in chronically violent neighborhoods. What limited research has been conducted indicates that children who are exposed to community violence are deeply affected by the experience (Bell & Jenkins, 1993; Martinez & Richters, 1993). Studies to date have reported that some children exposed to community violence–whether or not they themselves have been victimized–experience distress symptoms, including depression, anxiety, sleep problems, and impulsiveness (Freeman, Mokos, & Poznanski, 1993; Osofsky et al., 1993; Richters & Martinez, 1993). In relation to this, distress symptoms have been documented in children whose parents were victims of community violence, though the children did not witness the victimization (Dulmus & Wodarski, 2000), and family victimization, whether or not it was witnessed by the adolescent, was as strongly correlated with psychological distress as was personal victimization (Jenkins & Bell, 1994).

The reason that children are so deeply affected by the trauma of their parents may be because young children have limited cognitive abilities and make sense of their world through their focus on their primary caregiver(s). Children form attachments to primary caregivers and are emotionally and physically dependent on them. When a parent (primary caregiver) experiences a trauma, the child may be traumatized by the event related to their attachment to the parent. This is referred to as secondary trauma and is demonstrated through children's expression of related symptoms to a trauma that they did not witness (Figley, 1998).

The way children form attachments to parents differs by gender. Benenson, Morash, and Petrakos (1998) found that girls ages 4 to 5 are more emotionally involved with their mothers than were boys of the same age. This study also reported that girls enjoy being with their mothers more than boys (Benenson et al., 1998). Barber (1998) found that female children have a higher probability than male children of becoming insecurely attached following a divorce.

In addition to attachment differences, there is evidence that children differ by gender in their responses to trauma, violence and stress, as well. Studies that examined such differences have varying results. Two studies in 1991 found that, after disasters, girls report more symptoms of PTSD and other anxiety disorders than boys (Lonigan et al., 1991; Green et al., 1991). A study that examined the rates of depression and anxiety among bereaved children found that boys reported fewer depressive symptoms than girls up to 18 months after the death of a parent (Raveis, Seigel, & Karus, 1999). Leadbeater, Kupermine, Blatt, and Hertzog (1999) report gender differences in the internalizing and externalizing of problems relative to stressful life events; boys were at risk of externalizing their problems while girls tended to internalize. Cutler and Nolan-Hoeksema (1991) also suggest that girls are more likely to internalize problems than boys. Hoffman, Levy-Shiff, and Ushpiz (1993) evaluated gender differences among Israeli elementary school children in relation to stressful life events and found that increased anxiety and a trend towards heightened withdrawal was present in boys but not girls. Their findings further suggest that gender differences are correlated with the severity of the stressful events; as the severity of stress increased, boys' reactions were magnified.

A few studies indicate that there are gender differences in the psychological effects of trauma and violence on adolescents. Lipchitz and colleagues (1999) studied a group of inpatient adolescents and found that 93% of them had been exposed to a traumatic event such as community violence, family violence, or sexual abuse. Their results indicate that girls were more likely to develop post traumatic stress disorder (PTSD) from exposure to violence or traumatic events than boys, but boys with PTSD were more likely to have comorbid diagnoses of eating disorders, other anxiety disorders and somatization disorders. Furthermore, 72% of the girls in their sample had attempted suicide, whereas only 23% of the boys had made this attempt. Curle and Williams (1996) found clear gender differences in the psychological adjustment of adolescents, two years following a nearly fatal coach crash. They indicate that girls employed a larger variety of coping strategies and tended to describe such strategies as less effective at helping them cope than did boys. In addition, they found that girls reported higher symptoms of psychological distress and anxiety than boys.

The mentioned research, although inconsistent, suggests that there is a relationship between gender and children's reactions to trauma. This mounting evidence suggests that behavioral health treatments for children may need to be customized for gender.

CURRENT STUDY

In the authors' previous work (Dulmus & Wodarski, 2000), children, age 6-12 whose parents were victims of community violence (e.g., gunshot and stabbing victims), and whose victimization the children did not witness, were found to be experiencing distress symptoms related to their parents' victimization. The purpose of this current study is to do further analysis to examine children's psychological response to parental victimization by gender.

SAMPLE

The convenience sample consisted of 30 children, 6 through 12 years of age whose parent had been a victim of community violence. Data collection began in December 1997 and was completed in May 1998. Each consecutive admission into the trauma unit at the Erie County Medical Center (ECMC) in Buffalo, NY was screened and assessed over this six-month period to determine if they met the inclusion criteria until the 30 subjects were recruited for the study.

Inclusion criteria were as follows: (a) subjects had to be the biological children of parents victimized as a result of community violence; (b) the parents had to have received inpatient treatment (admitted to a medical floor for at least one night of stay) for related injuries at ECMC; (c) the child could not have witnessed their parents' victimization; and (d) the children could not have been currently receiving mental health services. Children with a documented history of mental retardation were excluded from the study. In addition, children whose parents were hospitalized due to domestic violence and/or self-inflicted wounds were also excluded from the study as these are not usually included in definitions of community violence.

METHODS

Data Collection Procedures

Thirty children whose parents had been victims of community violence serious enough to warrant inpatient treatment for subsequent injuries were recruited for this study. In addition to providing demographic information, parents completed an instrument to measure their children's distress symptoms. Information was obtained through interviews and self-administered instruments. All subjects were assured of the confidentiality of their responses. The primary investigator collected all data for this project at the Erie County Medical Center (ECMC). Data collection appointments were made for each participant 2 to 8 weeks following parents' victimization. The parents who completed the parent measures were the ones with whom the child resided. The primary investigator assisted the parents with completion of the parent measures as necessary. It took approximately one hour for each subject to complete his/her instrument package. All subjects were volunteers and were compensated with $20 cash.

Measures

A data collection form for parents to complete was developed for this study to collect sociodemographic information and other pertinent data. In addition, each parent completed the *Child Behavior Checklist* (Revised) (CBCL) (Achenbach, 1991). The CBCL is a 118-item checklist for parents to evaluate the behavior of their children 4 through 18 years of age and provides a total score and also scores for internalizing and externalizing behaviors. It asks questions regarding a wide variety of symptoms/behaviors their children may have experienced in the past six months and asks parents to respond to each question with three possible answers: "not true"; "somewhat true or sometimes true"; or "very true or often true." It is widely used and accepted in the field and has demonstrated good reliability and validity. The test-retest reliability of CBCL scale scores was supported by a mean test-retest ($r = .87$ for competency scales and $r = .89$ for problem scales over a seven-day period). Construct validity was supported by numerous correlates of CBCL scales, including significant associations with analogous scales on the Conner's *Parent Questionnaire*.

RESULTS

Sample Characteristics

All children were African American, with 47% being females. The mean age was 9.0 years. Though 67% percent of the children lived in single parent families, none lived exclusively with their fathers. The mean number of siblings in the home was 3.3, and the mean family gross income per month was $985. Children did not differ by previous violence exposure by gender. Additional characteristics included: Seventy-seven percent of parents who were victimized were males; of those, 77% had been shot and 23% had been stabbed. Their average length of stay in the hospital was 8.83 days with a standard deviation of 7.30. The minimum length of hospital stay was one night; the maximum stay was 24 nights. Fifty-seven percent of subjects had visited their injured parent while their parents were hospitalized. All subjects reported having had at minimum, monthly contact (by phone, in person, or a combination of the two) with their parents prior to victimization, with 61% reporting they had daily contact.

Statistical Analysis of CBCL by Gender

An independent t-test on the CBCL total score as reported by parent's of their children's distress symptoms showed no significant differences by gender [t (28) = 0.74, p > .464] (see Table 1). This test was followed up by an independent t-test on the CBCL externalizing score as reported by parents' of their children's distress symptoms which showed significant differences by gender for males [t (28) = 4.13, p < .001] (see Table 1) at the .05 level. An additional independent t-test on the CBCL internalizing score as reported by parents' of their children's distress symptoms showed no significant differences at the .05 level, but significance was found at the .10 level for females [t (28) = 1.65, p < .075] (see Table 1).

DISCUSSION

To date, significant differences in male and female adults' reactions to a tragic life event has been documented (Sprang & McNeil, 1998). The current study supports growing evidence that children exhibit such differences, as well. Findings of the present study suggest that children of parents who had been victims of community violence experienced dis-

TABLE 1. Child Behavior Checklist Scores (CBCL) by Gender

Group	n	m	sd	t	p
Total Score					
Male	16	45.4	17.0	0.74	.464
Female	14	41.1	13.7		
Externalizing Score					
Male	16	18.9	9.4	4.13	.001
Female	14	6.8	6.1		
Internalizing Score					
Male	16	11.7	7.2	1.82	.075
Female	14	16.9	8.3		

tress symptoms differently, depending on their gender. All children in the study were experiencing symptoms in the borderline clinical range as measured by the total score on the CBCL, with females having a mean score of 39.5 and males having a mean score of 38. The differences that were found by gender were in children's expression of symptoms, with females experiencing more internalizing symptoms (i.e., withdrawn, somatic complaints, anxiety, depression) and males experiencing more externalizing symptoms (i.e., aggression, delinquent behaviors). Such distinctions may be clinically useful when choosing approaches to intervention.

Other research indicates that boys restrict emotional expression, while girls increase emotional expression in adolescence (Polce-Lynch, Myers, Kilmartin, Forssmann-Falck, & Kliewer, 1998). Sigmon, Stanton, and Snyder (1995) found gender differences in coping, where females reported feeling less in control, feeling more stressed, and feeling more unpleasant towards dealing with certain situations as compared to men. The results of these studies that show gender differences in coping styles may help explain gender differences in children's responses to trauma that were found in the present study.

Feminist Perspective

The results of this study support the feminist theory perspective, which asserts that gender differences exist, due to multiple factors, such as socialization (Saulnier, 1996). It is important to briefly explain the basic premises of feminist theory and social work practice in order to relate feminist social work practice to the findings of this study.

The basic ideological framework of a feminist perspective is based upon several principles: (1) women are a special category with common characteristics such as biology and experience, (2) women should be the ones to define what is feminine, (3) feminism recognizes society is rooted in patriarchy, and (4) feminist perspective justifies a claim for root change to eliminate patriarchy (Ferree & Hess, 1994).

Feminist social work practice is based upon perspectives from feminist theory. Feminist social work practice is defined by Garvin and Reed (1995) as: "the action of developing, applying, reexamining, and revising feminist principles, which the practitioner can also use as guidelines for assessing and reflecting on practicing" (p. 42). Feminist therapy originated in the women's rights movement, and can be described as a philosophy of intervention rather than a set of techniques (Land, 1995), by which we interpret behavior according to the impact of emotional processes (Brown & Brodsky, 1992) and oppressive structures in the environment (Land, 1995). Feminist social workers and therapists hold the idea that theories of human behavior must be understood within the broader social context (Land, 1995). Feminist practice in social work suggests an analytical framework that is more fluid, with a multi-dimensional approach to problem solving and resolution based upon a relational context (Brandewein, 1987; Hyde, 1989) that recognizes gender differences. Consciousness raising, rethinking and reconceptualizing power are also central premises of feminist social work practice (Hyde, 1989).

Feminist social work practice emphasizes the need to include in interventions the experiences of women and people of both genders and all ages, races, ethnic backgrounds, classes, and sexual orientations (Land, 1995). Feminist practitioners also believe that their clients benefit from including a female clinician's experience as a woman, so elements of clinician self-disclosure are more heavily emphasized than in traditional psychotherapy; this is considered an important part of the empowerment process (Land, 1995). A feminist practice approach disputes the idea that nurturing characteristics in therapy are inappropriate or negative (Hyde, 1989). Based on the nurturing, inclusive emphasis of feminist practice, the authors conclude that feminist social work practice interventions are especially applicable when developing comprehensive social work services for children experiencing trauma-related distress, such as the children from the present study.

Feminist practitioners ascribe that mainstream psychoanalysis has mostly benefitted white heterosexual men in our society (Land, 1995), while ignoring children, women and people of color. However, feminist theory heavily emphasizes the role that social and cultural factors play on the socialized development of gender differences in boys and girls. Boudreau, Sennott, and Wilson (1986) indicate that sex labels assigned by parents and family are primarily responsible for gender identity in children.

The feminist social work practice approach is considered beneficial when working with women. The authors argue that children would also benefit from feminist social work interventions. Furthermore, feminist social work practice is based upon greater inclusiveness and an emphasis on client and clinician self disclosure, which may prove compatible with the therapeutic needs of children. Many feminist clinicians assume a gender blind stance that values the emotional worlds of both males and females, and many feminist practitioners stress gender sensitivity in working with families (Land, 1995). Because of its emphasis on inclusion and sensitivity to individual differences, the authors assert that feminist practice interventions would be appropriate for working with boys in addition to girls. Feminist practice advocates therapeutic techniques that recognize gender differences as an essential element in the client's response to therapy, which is extremely important in light of the findings of the current study.

The results of this study raise the question: What are the possible causes of the gender different responses to trauma in this study? A feminist social work perspective would argue that gender different relational patterns that children have with their parents result in girls taking different behavioral actions than boys (Gilligan, 1982; Land, 1995). For example, because girls are traditionally permitted to have intimate contact with mothers, they are socialized to behaviors that are more nurturing and cooperative (Gilligan, 1982; Land, 1995), which may explain their higher internalizing scores and other gender differences in relation to trauma.

Practice Recommendations

Feminist social workers need to come to a consensus on a definition of feminist practice that is widely accepted, and use that definition as a basis to develop and test models of practice based on feminist theory. Furthermore, empirical research needs to be conducted on feminist social work interventions with children, in order to build a knowledge base in the area of feminist theory and practice in relation to children, as the authors found no studies that examined the use of feminist techniques with children's interventions. Walker and Edwall (1987) indicate that family and children's issues would benefit from a feminist analysis of their problems and corresponding possible solutions. Although feminist social work therapists have begun to critique existing theories of family development (Land, 1995), more such critiques are necessary in order to discover the true benefits of a feminist approach to interventions that are responsive to gender difference in children. As McGoldrick and colleagues (1989) indicate, a therapist who is not conscious of the gender inequities embedded in our culture and is not trying to address these inequities in treatment, is contributing to the problems of families, and doing sexist family therapy.

It is essential that social workers are conscious about the existence of gender differences. Implications for practice might include social workers taking a feminist approach when working with traumatized children by providing assessment and interventions from a feminist perspective to address gender differences.

Limitations and Future Research

This study has a number of limitations. First, the design lacks random assignment. Second, the sample size is small (n = 30) and all persons in the study lived in the same area, which increases the risk of confounding variables and decreases generalizability, as certain results may be uniquely influenced by locale. Third, all findings were based on self-report data from parents; it is therefore possible that certain events and experiences were overestimated, underestimated or otherwise distorted through recall. Furthermore, all children in this sample were African-American. The sociodemographics of the sample limits the generalizability of the findings to all groups of children whose parents have been victimized.

Because this study did not control for confounding variables, this is considered beginning knowledge about non-witnessed parental victimization and distress in children as it varies by gender. More research needs to be done in other locales, with a larger sample size, greater age range and other racial backgrounds for results to be more conclusive. Studies need to be developed to examine the long-term effects of this type of trauma on children. It would be interesting to see if PTSD symptoms or other symptoms of mental illness develop in such children later in life. Additional research that examines how results vary by age and socioeconomic background, in addition to gender differences, would also be beneficial. Hoffman, Levy-Shiff, and Ushpiz (1993) suggest that more research needs to be done that controls for specific life stressors and their impact on gender and other variables. Although this study did control for the specific trauma of parental victimization, future research may want to focus on children's responses in relation to the gender of the parent who is victimized, as well as the type of parents' victimizations (i.e., beating, gunshot, stabbing) and circumstances surrounding the incidents as to the impact on children. Additional research needs to be conducted on different types of life stressors to assess if the severity of the stressor or trauma has an impact on children's responses by gender. In addition, a longitudinal study is recommended to determine any long-term outcomes for children whose parents have been victimized by community violence and how they might differ by gender.

This beginning knowledge may be helpful to clinicians when considering treatment approaches for children and for identifying groups of clients with similar problems for purposes such as group therapy and parent training groups (Achenbach, 1991). The study also indicates that clinicians may want to consider long-term treatment interventions that target children and their families to prevent adverse mental health reactions as a result of exposure to trauma. Treatment strategies need to respond to individual gender differences in the expression of symptoms related to trauma (Feiring, Taska, & Lewis, 1999).

The social work profession is historically rooted in feminist principles. Therefore, social work researchers need to take the lead in examining gender differences in all studies, while social work practitioners need to evaluate gender differences and the benefits of feminist practice techniques in response to such differences. This will allow for the development of empirically based gender sensitive interventions that will better meet the needs of the clients we serve, the majority of which are females (Morales & Sheafor, 1998).

REFERENCES

Achenbach, T. M. (1991). *Manual for the Child Behavior Checklist/4-18 and 1991 Profile*. Burlington, VT: University of Vermont Department of Psychiatry.

Barancik, J. (1983). Northeast Ohio trauma study. *American Journal of Public Health*, 73, 746-751.

Barber, N. (1998). Sex differences in dispostion towards kin, security of adult attachment, and sociosexuality as a function of parental divorce. *Evolution and Human Behavior, 19*, 125-132.

Bell, C. C., & Jenkins, E. J. (1993). Community violence and children on Chicago's southside. *Psychiatry, 56*, 46-54.

Benenson, J. F., Morash, D., & Petrakos, H. (1998). Gender differences in emotional closeness between preschool children and their mothers. *Sex Roles, 38*, 975-985.

Boudreau, F. A., Sennott, R. S., & Wilson, M. (1986). *Sex Roles and Social Patterns*. Praeger Publishers, New York.

Brandewein, R. A. (1987). Women and community organization. In D. S. Burden & N. Gottlieb (Eds.). *The Woman Client*. New York: Tavistock Publications.

Brown, L. S., & Brodsky, A. M. (1992). The future of feminist therapy. *Psychotherapy, 29*, 51-57.

Children's Defense Fund (1993). *Annual Report: The State of America's Children*. Washington DC: Author.

Curle, C. E., & Williams, C. (1996). Post-traumatic stress reactions in children: Gender differences in the incidence of trauma reactions at two years and examination of factors influencing adjustment. *The British Journal of Clinical Psychology, 35*, 297-309.

Cutler, S. E., & Nolen-Hoeksema, S. (1991). Accounting for sex differences in depression through female victimization: Childhood sexual abuse. *Sex Roles, 24*, 425-438.

Dulmus, C. N., & Wodarski, J. S. (2000). Trauma-related symptomatology among children of parents victimized by urban community violence. *American Journal of Orthopsychiatry, 70* (2), 272-277.

The Economist. (Oct. 3, 1998). Crime in America, 35-38.

Feiring, C., Taska, L., & Lewis, M. (1999). Age and gender differences in children's and adolescent's adaption to sexual abuse. *Child Abuse & Neglect, 23* (2), 115-128.

Ferree, M. M., & Hess B. B. (1994). *Controversy and Coalition: The New Feminist Movement Across Three Decades of Change*. New York: Twayne Publishers.

Figley, Charles R. (1998). *Burnout in families: The systemic costs of caring*. Boca Raton, FL: CRC Press.

Fingerhut, L., & Klienman, J. (1990). International and interstate comparisons of homicide among young males. *Journal of the American Medical Association, 263*, 3292-3295.

Freeman, L., Mokros, H., & Poznanski, E. (1993). Violent events reported by normal urban school-aged children: Characteristics and depression correlates. *Journal of the American Academy of Child and Adolescent Psychiatry, 32*, 419-423.

Garvin, C. D., & Reed, B. G. (1995). Sources and visions for feminist group work: Reflective processes, social justice, diversity and connection. In N. V. Bergh (Ed.), *Feminist Practice in the 21st Century* (pp. 41-69). Washington, DC: NASW Press.

Gilligan, C. (1982). *In a Different Voice*. Cambridge: Harvard University Press.

Green, B., Korol, M., Grace, M., Vary, M., Leonard, A., Gleser, G., & Smitson-Cohen, S. (1991). Children and disaster: Age, gender, and parental effects of PTSD symptoms. *Journal of the American Academy of Child and Adolescent Psychiatry, 30*, 945-951.

Harlow, C. (1989). *Injuries from Crime*: Bureau of Justice Statistics Special Report (#NCJ-116811). Washington, DC: Department of Justice, Bureau of Justice Statistics.

Hoffman, M., Levy-Shiff, R., & Ushpiz, V. (1993). Gender differences in the relation between stressful life events and adjustment among school-aged children. *Sex Roles, 29*, 441-455.

Hyde, C. (1989). A feminist model for macro-practice: Promises and problems. *Administration in Social Work, 13*, 145-181.

Jenkins, E. J., & Bell, C. C. (1994). Violence exposure, psychological distress and high risk behaviors among inner-city high school students. In S. Friedman (Ed.), *Anxiety Disorders in African Americans* (pp. 76-88). New York: Springer.

Land, H. (1995). Feminist clinical social work in the 21st century. In N. Van Den Bergh (Ed.) *Feminist Practice in the 21st Century* (pp. 3-19). Washington DC: NASW Press.

Leadbeater, B., Kupermine, G., Blatt, S., & Hertzog, C. (1999). A multivariate model of gender differences in adolescent's internalizing and externalizing problems. *Developmental Psychology, 35,* 1268-1282.

Lipschitz, D., Winegar, R., Hartnick, E., Foote, B., & Southwick, S. (1999). Posttraumatic stress disorder in hospitalized adolescents: Psychiatric comorbidity and clinical correlates. *Journal of the American Academy of Child and Adolescent Psychiatry, 38,* 385-392.

Lonigan, C., Shannon, M., Finch, A., Daughtery, T., & Taylor, C. (1991). Children's reactions to a natural disaster: Symptom severity and degree of exposure. *Advances in Behavior Research and Therapy, 13,* 135-154.

Lorion, R., & Saltzman, W. (1990). Children's exposure to community violence: Following a path from concern to research to action. In D. Reiss, J. E. Richters, M. Radke-Yarrow, & D. Scharff (Eds.), *Children and Violence* (pp. 55-65). New York: Guilford Press.

Manning, M. L., & Baruth, L. G. (1995). *Students at risk.* Boston: Allyn and Bacon.

Martinez, P., & Richters, J. (1993). The NIMH Community Violence Project II: Children's distress symptoms associated with violence exposure. *Psychiatry, 56,* 22-35.

McGoldrick, M., Anderson, C., & Walsh, F. (1989). *Women in Families: A Framework for Family Therapy.* New York: W.W. Norton.

Morales, A. T., & Sheafor, B. W. (1998). *Social Work: A profession of many faces.* Boston, MA: Allyn and Bacon.

Osofsky, J. S. (1995). The effects of exposure to violence on young children. *American Psychologist, 50* (9), 782-788.

Osofsky, J. D., Wewers, S., Hann, D. M., & Fick, A. C. (1993). Chronic community violence: What is happening to our children? *Psychiatry, 56,* 7-21.

Polce-Lynch, M., Myers, B. J., Kilmartin, C. T., Forssmann-Falck, R., & Kliewer, W. (1998). Gender and age patterns in emotional expression, body image, and self-esteem: A qualitative analysis. *Sex Roles, 38,* 1025-1048.

Raveis, V., Siegel, K., & Karus, D. (1999). Children's psychological distress following the death of a parent. *Journal of Youth and Violence, 28,* 165-180.

Richters, J. (1993). Community violence and children's development: Toward a research agenda for the 1990s. *Psychiatry, 56,* 3-6.

Richters, J. E., & Martinez, P. (1993). The NIMH Community Violence Project I: Children as victims of and witnesses to violence. *Psychiatry, 56,* 7-21.

Saulnier, C. (1996). *Feminist Theories and Social Work.* Binghamton, NY: The Haworth Press, Inc.

Sigmon, S. T., Stanton, A., & Snyder, C. R. (1995). Gender difference in coping: A further test of socialization and role constraint theories. *Sex Roles, 33,* 565-587.

Sprang, G., & McNeil, J. (1998). Post-homicide reactions: Grief mourning and post-traumatic stress disorder following a drunk driving fatality. *Omega, 37,* 41-58.

Walker, L. E. A., & Edwall, G. E. (1987). Domestic violence and determination of visitation and child custody in divorce. In D. J. Sonkin (Ed.), *Domestic Violence on Trial* (pp. 127-154). New York: Springer.

Protecting Children:
Exploring Differences and Similarities
Between Mothers
With and Without Alcohol Problems

Nancy J. Smyth
Brenda A. Miller
Pamela J. Mudar
David Skiba

SUMMARY. In this study, difficulties that women with alcohol problems and victimization experiences might have protecting their children from victimization were investigated. Mothers of children (ages 3-17)

Nancy J. Smyth, PhD, CSW, CASAH, and Brenda A. Miller are affiliated with the Center on Research on Urban Social Work Practice, University at Buffalo School of Social Work, The State University of New York.

Pamela J. Mudar is affiliated with the Research Institute on Addictions, Buffalo, NY.

David Skiba is affiliated with the University at Buffalo School of Social Work, The State University of New York.

Address correspondence to: Nancy J. Smyth, PhD, University at Buffalo School of Social Work, 685 Baldy Hall, Buffalo, NY 14216-1050 (E-mail: njsmyth@ buffalo.edu).

This research was supported by a grant from the National Institute on Alcohol Abuse and Alcoholism (Grant No. R01AA07554), PI: Dr. Miller, Co-PI, Dr. Smyth.

An earlier version of this paper was presented at the Society for Social Work and Research, January 2000, Charleston, SC.

[Haworth co-indexing entry note]: "Protecting Children: Exploring Differences and Similarities Between Mothers With and Without Alcohol Problems." Smyth, Nancy J. et al. Co-published simultaneously in *Journal of Human Behavior in the Social Environment* (The Haworth Social Work Practice Press, an imprint of The Haworth Press, Inc.) Vol. 7, No. 3/4, 2003, pp. 37-58; and: *Women and Girls in the Social Environment: Behavioral Perspectives* (ed: Nancy J. Smyth) The Haworth Social Work Practice Press, an imprint of The Haworth Press, Inc., 2003, pp. 37-58. Single or multiple copies of this article are available for a fee from The Haworth Document Delivery Service [1-800-HAWORTH, 9:00 a.m. - 5:00 p.m. (EST). E-mail address: docdelivery@haworthpress.com].

were recruited from a longitudinal study of women, alcohol problems, and victimization; women came from alcohol treatment programs, battered women's shelters, mental health clinics, drinking and driving programs, and a random household sample. Hypothetical parenting scenarios were constructed to assess mothers' ability to protect their children from victimization trauma. Women's responses to the scenarios were analyzed thematically and coded. Next, coded responses were analyzed quantitatively to identify significant differences among women with past alcohol and other drug (AOD) problems, current AOD problems, and no AOD problems. Women with current AOD problems were more likely than women with no AOD problems and women with past AOD problems to provide aggressive responses to scenarios. Women with past AOD problems were more likely than their non-addicted counterparts to perceive sexual abuse as a possibility, to attribute responsibility for the problem to the other participant only (seeing no role for their child), and to seek information about what happened from the other participant only. Findings suggest that some interpersonal problem-solving difficulties resolve when women become sober while others persist into recovery, potentially affecting women's ability to protect their children. *[Article copies available for a fee from The Haworth Document Delivery Service: 1-800-HAWORTH. E-mail address: <docdelivery@haworthpress. com> Website: <http://www.HaworthPress.com> © 2003 by The Haworth Press, Inc. All rights reserved.]*

KEYWORDS. Trauma, victimization, parenting, addiction

Under the best of circumstances, parenting effectively can be a challenge. Parents with alcohol and other drug (AOD) problems may face added difficulties in effectively meeting the needs of their children. Women with AOD problems, many of whom have childrearing responsibilities (Beckman & Amaro, 1986; Marsh & Miller, 1985), are no exception to this. As compared to women without AOD problems, these women are more likely to face limited personal and community resources, including inadequate income, problems with child care, and difficulty meeting needs for food, housing, transportation, and health care (Clayson, Berkowitz, & Brindis, 1995; Hawley, Halle, Drasin, & Thomas, 1995; Hermann et al., 1994; Marcenko, Spence, & Rohweder, 1994; Smyth & Miller, 1997). Limited resources may not only limit their ability to effectively meet children's needs but also may increase exposure to physical harm from others.

Given the high victimization rates among women with AOD problems (Miller & Downs, 1995; Miller, Downs, & Testa, 1993), and the suggestion by some researchers that victimization may be transmitted intergenerationally (e.g., Downs & Miller, 1996; Kantor, 1990; Lackey, 1995), the ability to protect children from victimization becomes a specific parenting concern for many addicted women. In this study we explored how women with AOD problems protect their children from victimization, as well as the ways in which their strategies for protection differed from women without AOD problems. A review of key concepts and findings that guided this research will place our findings in a larger context.

UNDERSTANDING INTERGENERATIONAL TRANSMISSION OF VICTIMIZATION

Women with AOD problems often have experienced childhood sexual abuse, childhood physical abuse, and adult victimization (Goldberg, 1995; Miller & Downs, 1995; Miller et al., 1993), experiences that can result in difficulty functioning effectively as a parent (Bernardi, Jones, & Tennant, 1989; Carson, Gertz, Donaldson, & Wonderlich, 1990; Smyth & Miller, 1997). These experiences have the potential to preclude a mother from sufficiently protecting her children from the harm presented by others, whether they be people inside or outside the family. For example, women with a history of childhood sexual abuse may be unable to provide buffers between their children and incestuous or physically abusive environments, thus posing a higher risk for victimization (Cole et al., 1992; Davis, 1990; Mian, Marton, LeBaron, & Birtwistle, 1994). Frequently these women are re-victimized as adults (Beitchman et al., 1992; Wyatt, Guthrie, & Notgrass, 1992). Patterns of re-victimization and intergenerational violence make it more difficult for women to protect their children. Beitchman and colleagues (1992) suggest several explanations for this intergenerational pattern, including: victimized children being forced out of the family into high-risk situations; the impact on self-esteem may make mothers conspicuous targets for sexually explosive men who may also abuse their children; women may idealize abusive men seeking to reestablish the special relationship with their father (when father was the source of abuse); and an impaired ability to identify correctly untrustworthy persons who may abuse their children.

A history of childhood physical or sexual abuse might also preclude a woman from learning appropriate parenting techniques, particularly related to protecting her own children from victimization. For women with histories of childhood victimization, insecure attachment to her parents becomes replicated as she mothers her own children (Alexander, 1992; Main & Goldwyn, 1984). Cole and Woolger (1989) reported that when fathers were the perpetrators of sexual abuse, women subsequently were more likely to use childrearing techniques that promoted extreme autonomy. Extreme autonomy may fail to promote sufficient protectiveness for children, thus making them vulnerable to violent victimization by others. For example, several studies have found that poor parental monitoring of adolescents' activities, including contacts with others, are associated with greater risk of a wide range of adolescent problem behaviors (Ary et al., 1999; Esbensen, Huizinga, & Menard, 1999; Forehand, Miller, Dutra, & Chance, 1997). These adolescent problem behaviors, in turn, increase the risk of victimization for adolescents (Esbensen et al., 1999; Windle, 1994).

Aspects of women's victimization history and childhood experiences may mediate the impact of maternal AOD on protecting children. For example, the type, severity, and frequency of abuse (Zuravin, McMillen, DePanfilis, & Risley-Curtis, 1996), or the quality of attachment relationships (Moncher, 1996), can affect the likelihood of transmission and might mediate the impact of AOD problems on protecting children. In addition, women with abusive partners may be unable to protect their children from violence by the partner (Stark & Flitcraft, 1988a, 1988b). Thus, the inability to protect children from violent victimization may be related to women's own ongoing victimization as well as their AOD problems.

UNDERSTANDING PROTECTIVENESS

Insight about mothers' protectiveness comes from studies that have examined what mothers do in response to their children's victimization. For example, a theoretical framework designed to assess protectiveness in cases of child sexual abuse included the following components: identification of a protecting adult from within the child's network; enabling this adult to protect all the children in the family by strengthening supports and resources; establishing important boundaries in the family, including removal of the perpetrator; support for maternal authority in the family; addressing the secrecy surrounding the child sexual abuse by informing siblings and extended family members to lessen the stigma for the child; and altering the network surrounding the child (Smith, 1995). In studying the protective and unprotective responses toward children victimized by violence, Faller (1988) reports a range of mothers' responses. Protective responses for children victimized by childhood sexual abuse (CSA) include calling the police or protective services, leaving the house with the children, making the perpetrator leave, and/or initiating divorce proceedings when the perpetrator is the partner/spouse, placing the child where the alleged perpetrator cannot have access to the child, and insisting the perpetrator get treatment. Unprotective responses included disbelieving the child, blaming the child, and continuing to expose the child to risky situations after the CSA and/or child abuse.

There is some research that suggests that mothers with AOD problems may have more difficulty protecting their children in comparison to other women. In one study among court cases for the protection of children, half had at least one caretaker with an alcohol and/or drug problem, and among those with a caretaker involved with alcohol or other drugs, 86% involved maternal substance abuse (Murphy et al., 1991). In an epidemiological sample of 673 mothers of children aged 8 to 11 years, Chilcoat and colleagues (1996) found that mothers' history of alcohol and drug abuse was associated with decreased levels of parental monitoring and supervision. Finally, Fleming and colleagues (1997) found that having an alcoholic mother was identified as a risk factor for girls being sexually abused by someone outside of the family.

Another confounding influence on maternal AOD problems and maternal protection of children may be women's own history of victimization. For example, one study found that incest survivors from alcoholic families were less consistent in their child rearing and made fewer age appropriate demands of their children than did both controls and adult children of alcoholics with no incest history (Cole, Woolger, Power, & Smith, 1992). What is not clear from this prior research is whether the relationship is due to mothers own AOD problems or whether the relationship is better explained by mothers' own victimization experiences.

This study addresses how women with AOD problems differ in the degree to which they protect their children from victimization. Based upon empirical evidence and clinical perspectives, it was hypothesized that women with AOD problems would experience more difficulty establishing protective parenting skills than would women without AOD problems. We also hypothesized that at least some of these difficulties would be less likely to occur if there was no current AOD use even when there had been prior AOD problems. However, because addicted women often have their own extensive histories of childhood and adult victimization, we expected some differences in protection strategies would remain even when women no longer had a current AOD problem. In addition, because little is known about protective parenting, part of this study's purpose was to define this concept more clearly. To achieve these aims, the study employed hypothetical scenarios that might involve risk to children.

METHOD

Sample and Procedure

This sample consists of a follow-up sample of individuals from a study originally designed to assess the relationships between a history of family violence and partner violence on the development of AOD-related problems (Miller et al., 1993).[1] The original sample consisted of 472 women between the ages of 18 and 45 years and was drawn from the following five sources: alcoholism outpatient treatment programs (n = 98), drinking driving classes for convicted offenders (n = 100), shelters for battered women (n = 97), outpatient mental health treatment programs (n = 77), and a random selection of households in the Buffalo, New York area (n = 100) (Miller & Downs, 1993; Miller et al., 1993; Miller & Downs, 1995). Data derived from this first interview are noted as T-1. A second interview (T-2) was conducted eighteen months later and included 416 women. The women included in these analyses represent those who completed a third follow up interview. During this wave (T-3), women with children between the ages 3 and 17 were identified and re-interviewed to assess the impact of mother's AOD problems and their ability to protect their children from victimization. A total of 246 of the original 472 women were identified as mothers of children aged 3 to 17 years, and nearly 70% (n = 171) of these mothers were interviewed in this third wave 3 (T-3). The average interval between wave 2 and wave 3 was two and one-half years.

The major criterion for inclusion in the present analyses was that the women have valid data on both the lifetime and current AOD use and AOD-related problem measures. This excluded one respondent for a final sample of 170.

The distribution of these respondents from the original five sources was as follows: 31 (18.2%) from alcoholism outpatient treatment programs, 17 (10.0%) from drinking driving classes for convicted offenders, 36 (21.2%) from shelters for battered women, 38 (22.4%) from mental health treatment programs, and 48 (28.2%) from the random household selection.

A structured interview, which contained both interviewer- and self-administered sections, was administered and required approximately two hours to complete. Women provided information about their children, and one child was randomly selected for inclusion in these analyses. Respondents were reimbursed for their time.

Measures

Mothers' AOD Problems (T1, T2, T3). Mothers' AOD problems were assessed through a variety of different measures. AOD-related problems in the lifetime based upon the DSM-III-R AOD dependence criteria (DIS; Robins et al., 1989) were assessed at the second interview. AOD-related problems during the past year (current) were reassessed in the third interview using this same measure. Regular drug[2] use (at least once a week for at least a month), daily drug use (for at least two weeks), and drug-related problems[3] (e.g., attempts to cut down, tolerance, withdrawal) were ascertained for the lifetime in interviews 1 and 2, and for the past year in interview 3. Mothers were categorized as having an AOD problem if they had any of the following: (1) three or more of the DSM-III-R diagnostic criteria for AOD dependence; (2) regular drug use and at least one drug-related problem; (3) no regular drug use, but two or more drug problems; or (4) daily drug use. For analytic purposes, mothers were divided into the following three groups based on when in their life they had an AOD problem: (1) Never; (2) Past–no current problems; or (3) Current–AOD problems in the last year.

Mothers' Protectiveness (T3). In order to assess mothers' protectiveness, hypothetical victimization risk scenarios were created so that information about alternate ways to conceptualize protection could be gathered. The scenarios included situations involving mothers' partners, a close family friend, extra-familial authority figures, and gangs. Mothers were asked to describe what they might do and how they might respond to each of the four scenarios for the child of focus. Mothers' responses were probed by trained interviewers in order to elicit the most detailed information. These scenarios were designed to be somewhat ambiguous without a clear cut determination of whether there had been a victimization incident. The purpose of these scenarios was to determine how the mother would "think through" the situation and respond to the incident. Content of scenarios are reported in the results section of this paper. Three different sets of age-appropriate scenarios were constructed for this study to reflect different types of victimization risks for children aged 3-7, 8-12, and 13-17. For children aged 13-17 years, two of the four scenario topics were gender-specific.

Thematic analyses of these scenarios were conducted according to the following procedure. A random sample of scenario transcripts from four or five mothers of children in each of the three age groups was first independently reviewed by the PI and Co-PI to identify and classify themes that represented mothers' responses and actions; then a coding scheme was developed, through consensus, to reflect the nine themes. Next, to test the coding scheme, the Co-PI and an independent qualitative analyst separately reviewed and coded a sample of the transcripts. Inter-rater reliability was high, over 90%. After minor modifications to the coding scheme (i.e., clarifications required during reliability checks), transcripts of all of the mothers responses to the scenarios were then reviewed and coded by the independent qualitative analyst.

For each mother, the presence or absence of each theme was coded. For eight of the themes, there was a simple categorization of present (1 point) or absent (0 points) for each scenario and the scores were then added across scenarios within the respective theme to provide an overall assessment of responding to scenarios on the identified themes. Thus, each woman could receive a range of 0 to 4 points for each of these themes (1 point × 4 scenarios). For one theme, "ability to explain the problem," three possible codes were possible (0 = no explanation; 1 = 1 explanation; 2 = multiple explanations). Thus, the sum for this item across the four scenarios ranged from 0-8 for each mother.

Comparisons of the summary scores from the thematic analyses across scenarios were then made across the three groups defined by mothers' AOD problem history: Never, Past, and Current, using analysis of variance (ANOVA). When results indicated significant differences across the groups ($p < .05$), the content of the excerpts extracted from the transcripts was carefully reviewed to determine possible explanations for these different scores. Excerpts that highlight the different responses across the groups are presented here.

RESULTS

For the total sample (n = 170), mothers ranged in age from 23 to 49; 32.9% were minorities, and about 30% were married at the time of the third interview. For the 170 children about whom the mothers reported, 31.2% were 3-7 years old; 40.6%, 8-12 years; 28.2%, 13-17 years) and nearly half (48.8%) were female. Ethnic data were comparable to the maternal data.

Women with (n = 105) and without (n = 65) a lifetime alcohol problem and women with (n = 30) and without (n = 140) a current alcohol problem were compared for demographic differences (see Table 1). Women with lifetime AOD problems, when compared to women without lifetime AOD problems, were significantly younger, of lower socioeconomic status, and less likely to be married. There were no differences between the groups with regard to race, or in the number of, or gender of, children at home. However, the children of mothers with lifetime AOD problems were, on average, slightly younger than those of the other mothers, probably a function of the mothers with AOD problems being younger. Characteristics were somewhat different for the mothers with current AOD problems when compared to mothers without current problems (see Table 1). While mothers with current AOD problems were younger than the other mothers and less likely to be married, they were not different in socioeconomic status or in the mean age of their children. They also were less likely than the mothers without current AOD problems to have male children. As with the mothers with lifetime AOD problems, the mothers with current AOD problems were not significantly different from their non-AOD problem peers with regard to their race or the number of children living at home.

Table 2 displays the victimization history by mothers' history of AOD problems. As reported in earlier findings (Miller et al., 1993; Miller & Downs, 1993, 1995), mothers with lifetime AOD problems reported a significantly higher prevalence of childhood and adulthood victimization than did the mothers without lifetime problems. Specifically, mothers with AOD problems reported more childhood sexual abuse, childhood severe maternal and paternal physical abuse, severe partner violence, and non-sexual adult victimization. These differences were not evident when comparing mothers with and without current AOD problems, although this may be a function of inadequate power resulting from the small number of cases reporting current AOD problems (n = 30) and the inclusion of the women with prior AOD problems in the "no current" AOD problems category.

Protectiveness Results. In Table 3, the nine themes identified in the interview transcripts are presented: (1) explanation or conceptualization of what might be happening in the incident; (2) sources for information gathering; (3) style of gathering information; (4) attribution of responsibility for incident; (5) considered sex abuse as occurring; (6) considered physical abuse as occurring; (7) considered alcohol/drugs as involved;

(8) identification of plan of action; and (9) nature of mother's hypothesized reactions.

Briefly, these themes can be described as follows. Explanation/conceptualization addresses the possible causes of the scenario that are offered by women. Information sources considers to whom mothers turn to gather necessary information to determine what is happening or what to do about the problem. Information style considers how women asked for information (e.g., asking questions in a manner that conclusions

TABLE 1. Sample Characteristics by Mothers' History of Alcohol Problems

	Lifetime Alcohol Problems			Current Alcohol Problems		
	Yes	No	$t_{(df)}$ or $\chi^2_{(df)}$	Yes	No	$t_{(df)}$ or $\chi^2_{(df)}$
Mothers' Characteristics	(N = 105)	(N = 65)		(N = 30)	(N = 140)	
Age (years)	35.4±5.6	39.0±5.8	$-4.03^{***}{}_{(168)}$	33.7±5.8	37.5±5.8	$-3.23^{**}{}_{(168)}$
Socioeconomic Status (SES)	28.0±13.5	34.7±15.3	$-2.86^{**}{}_{(164)}$	26.9±12.3	31.3±14.9	$-1.71_{(164)}$
Number of Children at Home	1.8±1.2	2.2±1.2	$-1.89_{(168)}$	1.6±1.0	2.0±1.2	$-1.91_{(168)}$
Married (%)	21.0	45.3	$11.20^{***}{}_{(1)}$	10.0	43.5	$7.05^{**}{}_{(1)}$
Minority (%)	33.3	32.2	$0.02_{(1)}$	46.7	30.0	3.11(1)
Child Characteristics						
Age (years)	9.2±4.3	10.9±4.3	$-2.59_{(164)}{}^{*}$	8.8±4.4	10.1±4.3	$-1.47_{(168)}$
Male (%)	54.3	46.2	$1.06_{(1)}$	33.3	55.0	$4.64_{(1)}{}^{*}$

[1]mean ± standard deviation or percent
*p < .05; **p < .01; ***p < .001

TABLE 2. Mothers' Victimization History[1] by Mothers' History of Alcohol Problems

	Lifetime Alcohol			Current Alcohol Problems		
	Yes	No	$t_{(df)}$ or $\chi^2_{(df)}$	Yes	No	$t_{(df)}$ or $\chi^2_{(df)}$
Victimization History	(N = 105)	(N = 65)		(N = 30)	(N = 140)	
Childhood Sexual Abuse (%)	62.9	26.2	$21.65^{***}{}_{(1)}$	56.7	47.1	$0.90_{(1)}$
Childhood Maternal Severe Violence	0.9±1.1	0.5±0.9	$2.40^{*}{}_{(168)}$	0.9±1.1	0.7±1.0	$1.14_{(168)}$
Childhood Paternal Severe Violence	1.0±1.5	0.4±0.9	$3.11^{**}{}_{(166)}$	0.7±1.3	0.8±1.3	$-0.33_{(166)}$
Severe Partner Violence (%)	62.9	36.9	$10.84^{**}{}_{(1)}$	66.7	50.0	$2.75_{(1)}$
Non-Sexual Adult Victimization (%)	60.0	38.5	$7.64^{**}{}_{(1)}$	60.0	50.0	$0.99_{(168)}$

[1]mean ± sd or percent
*p < .05; **p < .01; ***p < .001

TABLE 3. Mothers' Protectiveness Scenario Responses by Mothers' History of Alcohol Problems (n = 170)

Scenario Theme (possible range of scores)	Maternal AOD Status			F	df
	Never (n = 65)	Past only (n = 75)	Current (n = 30)		
Ability to explain problem (0-8)	4.4±1.3	4.6±1.5	3.9±1.8	2.46+	(2, 158)
Information source					
Child only (0-4)	1.3±0.9	1.2±1.0	1.1±0.9	0.67	(2, 165)
Other participant only (0-4)	0.1±0.4$_a$	0.5±0.8$_b$	0.4±0.7	3.76*	(2, 165)
Both (0-4)	1.3±1.1	1.3±1.2	1.0±0.9	1.22	(2, 165)
Consider sexual abuse (0-4)	1.1±1.0$_a$	1.6±1.1$_b$	1.5±1.3	4.05*	(2, 163)
Consider physical abuse (0-4)	1.4±1.0	1.6±1.1	1.4±1.1	1.05	(2, 163)
Attribution of responsibility					
Child only (0-4)	0.5±0.7	0.3±6.0	0.4±0.8	1.58	(2, 165)
Other participant only (0-4)	1.8±1.3$_a$	2.4±1.2$_b$	2.0±1.0	4.13*	(2, 165)
Both (0-4)	1.2±1.0	0.9±1.0	0.9±0.8	1.04	(2, 165)
Child only (0-4)	0.5±0.7	0.3±6.0	0.4±0.8	1.58	(2, 165)
Suggests alcohol involvement (0-4)	0.2±0.5	0.1±0.4	0.0±0.2	1.25	(2, 165)
Information seeking from child					
Sought no info (0-4)	0.9±1.0	1.0±1.1	1.3±1.1	1.25	(2, 164)
Suggested concerns (0-4)	0.8±0.8	0.8±0.9	0.6±0.7	0.79	(2, 164)
Asked in other way (0-4)	1.1±1.1	1.0±1.0	0.9±0.9	0.28	(2, 164)
Information seeking from other participant					
Sought no info (0-4)	2.0±1.4	1.7±1.4	1.9±1.4	0.48	(2, 165)
Suggested concerns (0-4)	0.4±0.7	0.6±0.7	0.5±0.8	0.83	(2, 165)
Ask in other way (0-4)	0.4±0.6	0.4±1.7	0.2±0.4	1.05	(2, 165)
Plan of action identified (0-4)	2.6±1.1	3.0±0.9	2.8±1.2	2.82+	(2, 164)
Mother's strong emotions (0-4)	0.1±0.3$_a$	0.3±0.6	0.5±0.8$_b$	4.37*	(2, 165)
Mother's upset with child (0-4)	0.1±0.4	0.5±0.3	0.1±0.2	0.28	(2, 165)
Mother's aggressive response (0-4)	0.2±0.5$_a$	0.2±0.5$_a$	0.6±0.9$_b$	4.69*	(2, 165)

Note: Mean SD unadjusted. Groups with different subscripts are significantly different (p < .05). Tukey adjustment for multiple comparisons. Df = degrees of freedom. Each theme element was coded as absent (0) or present (1), with the exception of the first theme, "ability to explain the problem" which was coded as none (0), one explanation (1), multiple explanations (2). Because each mother was presented with four scenarios, responses could range from 0-4 for all theme elements, except for "ability to explain the problem," which could range from 0-8.
+ p < .10; *p < .05

about what happened, asking open-ended questions, etc.). Attribution of responsibility addressed whom mothers held responsible for the problem situation, the child, the other person, or both. Considering physical abuse, sexual abuse, or alcohol and drugs, each determined whether or not mothers offered theses possible factors as playing a role in the scenario. Identification of a plan of action described what, if any, course of action women proposed. Nature of response examined the emotional character of the mothers' proposed actions, e.g., strong emotions and the use of aggression or intimidation.

To explore whether there were differences in the identification of these themes across the three groups (no prior alcohol problems, past only, and current alcohol problems), a series of ANOVAs were performed. Significant differences emerged on four themes: sources for information gathering, attribution of responsibility, considered sexual abuse as occurring, and nature of mother's reactions. These four themes are discussed more fully and excerpts are provided to illustrate the differences between mothers' responses based upon their status of AOD use.

Sources for Information Gathering. Ideally, effective problem-solving involves seeking out information from as many sources as possible. In this theme, mothers identified the person from whom they would seek information in order to decide what the problem was and the appropriate action. Responses could be coded into three major categories: seeking information from children only, seeking information from the other person identified as involved in the incident; and seeking information from both. When compared to mothers without AOD problems, AOD mothers (Past and Current) more often identified going only to the other person, and not the child, to gather information about the problem. The following scenario and responses illustrate these differences.

> Scenario A (3-7 year olds): Suppose you left (child) in the care of your older daughter. Afterward, you noticed bruises on (child's) back and when you touched her/him s/he backed away. Since then (child) has been unusually quiet, hanging onto you wherever you go and doesn't want you to leave her/him alone with her/his sister. What, if anything, would you do?

Current Mom: I'd beat her butt. The older sister. Ask her what the hell happened. Probably start hitting her, honestly. (10613-01)

Never Mom: I'd first ask (Child) what happened and then I'd ask her older sister what happened . . . I'd sit them both down together and I'd find out between the two of them what happened. (20093-2)

Past Mom: I would confront his sister and ask her what happened, how he got the bruises. Then I would take it from there depending on what her response was. Obviously he must have gotten the bruises while he was in her care . . . (40693-4)

Attribution of Responsibility. In addition to differences in information gathering, there were differences that emerged in the attribution of responsibility for the problem situation. Mother's assessments of who was responsible for creating the problem were captured by three categories, the child, the other person, or both. Past AOD Mothers were most likely to attribute responsibility to the other person in the scenario. The responses to Scenario A from a Past Mother (4069-4) illustrate the implied attribution of responsibility to the other person only. A contrasting response from a Never Mother to Scenario B follows and illustrates attribution of responsibility to both parties:

Never Mom: Maybe they were playing too rough and she (Child) fell down. (20093-2)

Responses to the following scenario provide some additional illustrations of these differences.

Scenario B (13-17 year olds): Suppose that last week (child) and your partner got into a shoving match over (child's) coming home late from a friend's house. (Child) got bruised. Your partner says he is getting fed up and if (child) doesn't start listening to him he is really going to show (child) who's boss. What, if anything, would you do?

Past Mom: He would have to leave. I would tell him it's time for you to go. Call 911 to remove him if he wouldn't leave. He's trying to dominate the household. (10993)

Never Mom: Again, I'd be the mediator. Normally, I would speak . . . again, my husband is not a volatile person, but if he were, I would number one try to speak to him about his outburst first. Then I would, of course, dialog with (Child) about the importance of being home on time and that we have rules in this family, this doesn't please your father to do such and such. But first I would not allow the hitting I don't think. (50283-1)

Suggesting Sexual Abuse as an Explanation. In addition to attributional differences, mothers differed in the frequency with which they identified sexual abuse as a possible explanation for what was happening in a given scenario. This theme emerged from examination of the possible explanations offered for various scenarios. Mothers with Past AOD problems were more likely than Never Mothers to suggest sexual abuse as a possible explanation for a problem scenario. (Current Mothers were almost as likely as Past Mothers to identify this explanation, but the differences were not significant.) These differences can be contrasted in examining responses to the following scenario involving a teacher.

> Scenario C (8-12 year olds): Suppose that (child) has a favorite teacher she is always talking about. (Child) was chosen as the teacher's "special helper" and has been staying after school alone with the teacher. Last week (child) came home later than usual and seemed upset. The next day (child) announced she doesn't like her teacher anymore and wants to stop being the "special helper."

Never Mom: I would try and ask (daughter) if there was something that happened between her and the teacher and try and make her feel that she could talk to me about it. Then if it was something that the teacher did, I would confront the teacher . . .

Interviewer: What do you think is going on here?

Never Mom: I would hope just a communication problem and nothing more. (50673-3)

A mother with Past AOD problems responded to this same scenario in the following way:

Past Mom: Ask (son) what happened first. Would never have son go back there again. Second, confront the teacher ask, "What would cause (son) to react this way?" Maybe this was sexual or physical abuse. It'd be strange for my son to react that way as he usually likes everyone. Strange behavior would be a red flag. (50183)

Nature of Mother's Response: Emotional and Aggressive Responses. Mothers with current AOD problems were most likely to react to scenarios with strong emotional responses, and to offer problem-solving strategies that utilized violence or intimidation.

> Scenario D (8-12 year olds): Imagine that (child) and her older brother have been having problems getting along. You've noticed

bruises and cuts on (child) when they've been left alone together. Last week (child) had a black eye and wouldn't tell you what had happened. Since then (child) doesn't come home from school until she knows you are home, and doesn't want to be left alone with her brother.

Current Mom: I'd probably ask him and then I'd kill him (laughs) . . . I'd probably jump on him and beat the crap out of him if he did that. I'm sure I would. Not kill him kill him, but give him a taste of his own medicine. (30783-1)

Another mom's response to the teacher scenario presented earlier provides a further example:

Current Mom: I'd be down to that school questioning that teacher in a heartbeat.

Interviewer: What kinds of things would you say to the teacher?

Current Mom: "What did you do to my son?" Stuff like that really makes me think.

Interviewer: What do you mean "stuff like that?"

Current Mom: First thing that would pop into my head if he ever came home like that would be that teacher did something to him that he did not like at all.

Interviewer: Like what?

Current Mom: Probably touched him in the wrong way or made him do something that he didn't want to do. I don't know. I'd kill him.

Interviewer: What do you mean by "kill him?"

Current Mom: Pow-pow right between the eyes. Nobody gonna mess with my son. I know I shouldn't be sounding like this but he was my first born and he's my little pride and joy. I would never let anybody hurt him, never. (30303-1)

In contrast, Never Mothers were more likely to respond to situations with lower intensity, and less aggressive emotional responses. For example, in response to the teacher scenario (C) above, this Never Mother states:

Try to get out of (daughter) how can somebody that she likes all of a sudden . . . what happened that turned her against this person so fast? If I didn't have any response with that, I would go the teacher and explain what I [had] noticed with (daughter) and the sudden change and why . . . the sudden change. What might be the cause of this sudden change? . . . (40723-4)

Interestingly, Past AOD Mothers were also less likely to provide aggressive responses. For example, this mother responded to the scenario presented earlier involving the partner (Scenario B) as follows:

He (partner) would have to leave. I would tell him it's time for you to go. Call 911 to remove him if he wouldn't leave. He's trying to dominate the household. (10993)

DISCUSSION

Differences in protectiveness were found in responses to protection scenarios for mothers with both past and current AOD problems when compared to mothers with no AOD problems. However, most differences were identified between mothers with past AOD problems and those with no history of AOD problems. Although almost no differences were identified between mothers with current AOD problems (except with the use of aggression) and the other groups, this may be due to low power resulting from the small sample of current AOD mothers. In fact, many of the responses appear to be similar between mothers with past and current AOD problems.

Further replication of these findings are needed with additional samples. In addition, it is possible that the methodology employed, that is, presenting participants with hypothetical scenarios, generates responses that have no relationship to what participants would do in actual situations. With these limitations in mind, possible interpretations of the findings are described below. Clearly, all of these offered interpretations would need to be subject to further investigation.

Mothers with current AOD problems were more likely than Never mothers to respond with strong emotional reactions and more likely that Past and Never mothers to suggest aggressive responses to problems. This is not surprising given that alcohol, in particular, is known to increase the potential emotional volatility and violence (e.g., see Galanter, 1997). The lack of difference between the Past and Never mothers on this factor suggests that sobriety alone may resolve some of this difficulty.

However, in separate analyses with these same women (Miller, Smyth, & Mudar, 1999), we found that mothers with past AOD problems still have higher levels of punitiveness than mothers with no history of AOD problems. Taken together, these findings suggest that while some aspects of aggressiveness may decrease in sobriety, that not all of these behaviors resolve with addiction treatment.

Mothers with past history of AOD problems differed from the mothers with no AOD history in several ways. They were more likely to seek information about what had happened from only the other participant (instead of the child only, or both participants). This suggests that some family communication problems may persist well into recovery. In addition, seeking information from the other participant only probably does not do much to promote open communication between a mother and her (potentially) victimized child, perhaps decreasing mothers' abilities to protect their children.

Past AOD mothers also were more likely to *only* attribute responsibility for a problem to the other participant, instead of the child or both parties. A couple of explanations for this come to mind. It is possible that these mothers' own victimization history leads them to hold other participants more responsible in general. Or perhaps mothers with past AOD problems harbor some guilt about the impact of their AOD use on their children, and so avoid seeing that their children are behaving in a way that suggests they might have any problems. If the latter is true, then mothers may well miss the emergence of problems in their children (i.e., AOD problems, delinquency) until these problems get extreme; this would limit their ability to intervene early.

Another important finding was that mothers with Past AOD problems were more likely than mothers with no AOD problems to perceive sexual abuse as the problem. This suggests that their own abuse experiences may contribute to hyper-vigilance towards their children on this issue. Although this sensitization towards a possible problem may be positive, it is also possible that seeing sexual abuse risk everywhere makes it more difficult for mothers to distinguish more serious risk situations. It is worth noting that untreated trauma/posttraumatic stress disorder (PTSD) is associated with a pervasive sense of fear and an inability to distinguish current threats from feelings of threat associated with unhealed trauma, as well as a tendency to view neutral stimuli as threatening (van der Kolk, 1996); so, this finding may indicated the presence of untreated PTSD among Past Mothers.

Implications for Human Behavior Knowledge

These results may shed some light on the complex phenomena of the intergenerational transmission of AOD problems and victimization in families, at least in those cases where mothers have addiction problems. It would appear that while some problems in parenting, such as overly emotional and aggressive responses, might relate directly to the effects of heavy use of AOD, other problems might have their origins in the life experiences of the mothers. Mothers' extensive victimization history may offer them inadequate opportunities to learn effective interpersonal problem-solving. Moreover, the impact of victimization may be evident in the perceptions about responsibility and victimization risk that mothers bring to parenting. These perceptions, or schema, might then influence (or limit) mothers' recognition of the options and choices available to them in any particular situation.

Implications for Practice

Our findings suggest that mothers with AOD problems experience problems with interpersonal problem-solving and communication. While some problems remit after mothers stop drinking (and receive treatment), it appears that this may not be true for others. Poor family communication is associated with the risk of the development of a range of problems in youth including AOD problems and delinquency (Deren, 1986; Malinosky-Rummell, 1993; Polusny & Follette, 1995); in addition, poor communication cannot help mothers protect their children from victimization. Finally, family communication problems can only place more strain on a woman in recovery who is trying to regain control over her life. These findings suggest the need for AOD treatment agencies to add family communication components to their programs. Although it is possible to refer women to other agencies for such programs, providing comprehensive treatment within a setting may reduce strain on the woman and her family. In addition, general parenting and family communication programs cannot adequately address the guilt and shame associated with parenting issues for women with AOD problems (Smyth & Miller, 1997).

Our findings also suggest that mothers' own childhood sexual abuse experiences may influence mothers' perceptions of potential sexual abuse of their children in various scenarios. This may serve a protective function for their children. However, it is also possible that these mothers will have difficulty distinguishing between low and high risk victimization risk situations, a characteristic that can be associated with untreated PTSD. While this point merits further research, it does suggest that treatment of trauma among addicted women could serve to help mothers identify moderate to high risk sexual abuse situations threatening their own children. In addition, it would seem prudent to include modules on sexual abuse risk in parenting programs for mothers with AOD problems.

These recommendations serve to highlight an important point: appropriate treatment of addicted mothers is an appropriate first step in a comprehensive prevention program for their children, a population known to be at risk of a wide range of problems (Deren, 1986; Malinosky-Rummell, 1993; Polusny & Follette, 1995). If we are to interrupt the intergenerational cycle of addiction and victimization, treatment of mothers with AOD problems needs to move beyond just treating the AOD problems to treating the whole person in the context of her social relationships.

NOTES

1. NIAAA Grant No. RO1AA07554 awarded to Dr. Brenda A. Miller.

2. Use and problem information about the following drug classes was ascertained in the third interview: sedatives/tranquilizers, stimulants, analgesics, inhalants, hallucinogens, marijuana/hashish, cocaine, and heroin/methadone. In interviews 1 and 2, the drug classes included: barbiturates, tranquilizers, amphetamines, marijuana/hashish, crack, cocaine, heroin, other opiates, psychedelics, and other drugs.

3. At interview 1, problem measures included both drug-specific items (i.e., dependence, attempts to cut down, tolerance, withdrawal, health problems, family/social/work/school/police problems, emotional/psychological problems) and global items about drug problems (i.e., telling a doctor about problems with drugs, telling another professional, taking medication more than once, frequent interference with life or activities. At interview 2, two global drug problems questions were asked. One about ever feeling dependent, wanting to cut down and could not, feeling the need for larger amount to get high, or withdrawal symptoms, and the other about being unable to attend to work or household duties, having legal problems, or health problems due to drugs. At interview 3, questions about attempting to cut down, tolerance, and withdrawal symptoms were asked about each of the drugs used in the last year.

REFERENCES

Aiken, L. S., & West, S. G. (1991). *Multiple regression: Testing and interpretation interactions.* Newbury Park, CA: Sage Publications.

Alexander, P. C. (1992). Application of attachment theory to the study of sexual abuse. *Journal of Consulting and Clinical Psychology, 60,* 185-195.

Ary, D. V., Duncan, T. E., Biglan, A., Metzler, C. W., Noell, J. W., & Smolkowski, K. (1999). Development of adolescent problem behavior. *Journal of Abnormal Child Psychology, 27(2)*, 141-150.

Beckman, L. J., & Amaro, H. (1986). Personal and social difficulties faced by women and men entering alcoholism treatment. *Journal of Studies on Alcohol, 47*, 135-145.

Beitchman, J. H., Zucker, K. J., Hood, J. E., DaCosta, G. A., Akman, D., & Cassavia, E. (1992). A review of the long-term effects of child sexual abuse. *Child Abuse and Neglect, 16*, 101-118.

Bernardi, E., Jones, M., & Tennant, C. (1989). Quality of parenting in alcoholics and narcotic addicts. *British Journal of Psychiatry, 154*, 677-682.

Blume, S. B. (1991). Children of alcoholic and drug-dependent parents. In P. Roth (Ed.), *Alcohol and Drugs are Women's Issues* (Vol. 1, pp. 166-172). Metuchen, NJ: Women's Action Alliance and The Scarecrow Press.

Carson, D. K., Gertz, L. M., Donaldson, M., & Wonderlich, S. A. (1990). Family-of-origin characteristics and current family relationships of female adult incest victims. *Journal of Family Violence, 5*, 153-171.

Clayson, Z., Berkowitz, G., & Brindis, C. (1995). Themes and variations among seven comprehensive perinatal drug and alcohol abuse treatment models. *Health & Social Work, 20*, 234-238.

Cohen, J., & Cohen, P. (1983). *Applied multiple regression/correlation analysis for the behavioral sciences*, 2nd ed. Hillsdale, NJ: Erlbaum.

Cole, P. M., & Woolger, C. (1989). Incest survivors: The relation of their perceptions of their parents and their own parenting attitudes. *Child Abuse and Neglect, 13*, 409-416.

Cole, P. M., Woolger, C., Power, T. G., & Smith, K. D. (1992). Parenting difficulties among adult survivors of father-daughter incest. *Child Abuse and Neglect, 16*, 239-249.

Davis, S. K. (1990). Chemical dependency in women: A description of its effects and outcome on adequate parenting. *Journal of Substance Abuse Treatment, 7*, 225-232.

Downs, W. R., & Miller, B. A. (1996). Inter-generational links between childhood abuse and alcohol-related problems. In L. Harrison (Ed.), *Alcohol Problems and Community Care* (pp. 15-51). London: Routledge Ltd.

Elliott, D. (1989). *Denver Youth Survey Parent Interview Schedule*. Institute of Behavioral Science, Denver Youth Survey: University of Colorado.

Esbensen, F. A., Huizinga, U., & Menard, S. (1999). Family content and criminal victimization in adolescence. *Youth & Society, 31(2)*, 168-198.

Faller, C. K. (1988). *Child sexual abuse: An interdisciplinary manual for diagnosis, case management, and treatment*. New York: Columbia University Press.

Finkelstein, N. (1994). Treatment issues for alcohol- and drug-dependent pregnant and parenting women. *Health & Social Work, 19*, 7-15.

Forehand, R., Miller, K. S., Dutra, R., & Chance, M. W. (1997). Role of parenting in adolescent deviant behavior: Replication across and within two ethnic groups. *Journal of Consulting & Clinical Psychology, 65(6)*, 1036-1041.

Galanter, M. (Ed.). (1997). *Recent developments in alcoholism, vol. 13: Alcohol and violence-epidemiology, neurobiology, psychology, family issues*. New York: Plenum.

Goldberg, M. E. (1995). Substance-abusing women: False stereotypes and real needs. *Social Work, 40,* 789-798.

Hawley, T. L., Halle, T. G., Drasin, R. E., & Thomas, N. G. (1995). Children of addicted mothers: Effects of the "crack epidemic" on the caregiving environment and the development of preschoolers. *Amercian Journal of Orthopsychiatry, 65(3),* 364-379.

Hermann, J., Shur, G., McKinney, S., Fields, C., & Sambrano, S. (1994, May). *Implementation evaluation findings from substance abuse treatment programs for pregnant and parenting women.* Paper presented at the American Psychological Association's National Multidisciplinary Conference on Psychosocial and Behavioral Factors in Women's Health: Creating an Agenda for the 21st Century, Washington, DC.

Jaccard, J., Turrisi, R., & Wan, C. K. (1990). *Interaction effects in multiple regression.* Newbury Park, CA: Sage.

Kantor, G. K. (1990, August). *Parental drinking, violence, and child aggression: A multi-generational model of family violence.* Paper presented at the meeting of the American Psychological Association. Boston, MA.

Lackey, C. (1995). *Controlling the intergenerational transmission of partner abuse.* Boulder, CO: University of Colorado.

Lozina, C., Russell, M., & Mudar, P. (1995). Correlates of alcohol-related problems in African-American and white gynecologic patients. *Alcoholism: Clinical and Experimental Research, 19* (1), 25-30.

Main, M., & Goldwyn, R. (1984). Predicting rejection of her infant from mother's representation of her own experience: Implications for the abused-abusing intergenerational cycle. *Child Abuse and Neglect, 8,* 203-217.

Marcenko, M. O., Spence, M., & Rohweder, C. (1994). Psychosocial characteristics of pregnant women with and without a history of substance abuse. *Health & Social Work, 19,* 17-22.

Marsh, J. C., & Miller, N. A. (1985). Female clients in substance abuse treatment. *The International Journal of the Addictions, 20,* 995-1019.

Mian, M., Marton, P., LeBaron, D., & Birtwistle, D. (1994). Familial risk factors associated with intrafamilial and extrafamilial sexual abuse of three- to five-year-old girls. *Canadian Journal of Psychiatry, 39,* 348-353.

Miller, B. A., & Downs, W. R. (1995). Violent victimization among women with alcohol problems. In M. Galanter (Ed), *Recent developments in alcoholism, Vol. 12: Alcoholism and women.* (pp. 81-101). New York: Plenum Publishing Corporation.

Miller, B. A., & Downs, W. R. (1993). The impact of family violence on the use of alcohol by women. *Alcohol Health and Research World, 17* (2), 137-143.

Miller, B. A., Downs, W. R., & Testa, M. (1993). Interrelationships between victimization experiences and women's alcohol use. *Journal of Studies on Alcohol, Supplement No. 11,* 109-117.

Miller, B. A., Smyth, N. J., & Mudar, P. J. (1999). Mother's alcohol and other drug problems and their punitiveness toward their children. *Journal of Studies on Alcohol, 60,* 632-642.

Moncher, F. J. (1996). The relationship of maternal adult attachment style and risk of physical child abuse. *Journal of Interpersonal Violence, 11* (3), 335-350.

Murphy, J. M., Jellinek, M., Quinn, D., Smith, G., Poitrast, F. G., & Goshko, M. (1991). Substance abuse and serious child mistreatment: Prevalence, risk, and outcome in a court sample. *Child Abuse and Neglect, 15,* 197-211.

Reed, B. G. (1985). Drug misuse and dependency in women: The meaning and implications of being considered a special population or minority group. *The International Journal of the Addictions, 20,* 13-62.

Robins, L., Helzer, J., Cottler, L., & Goldring, E. (1989). NIMH diagnostic interview schedule: Version III revised (DIS-III-R). St. Louis, MO: Washington University.

Skinner, H. A. (1979). *Lifetime drinking history: Administration and scoring guidelines.* Toronto: Addiction Research Foundation.

Smyth, N. J., & Miller, B. A. (1997). Parenting issues for women with alcohol and other drug problems. In S. L. A. Straussner & E. Zelvin (Eds.), *Gender issues in addiction* (pp. 123-150). New York: Jason Aronson.

Straus, M. A. (1979). Measuring intrafamily conflict and violence: The Conflict Tactics (CT) scales. *Journal of Marriage and the Family, 41,* 75-88.

van der Kolk, B. A. (1996). The body keeps the score: Approaches to the psychobiology of posttraumatic stress disorder. In B. A. van der Kolk, A. C. McFarlane, & L. Weisaeth (Eds.), *Traumatic stress* (pp. 214-241). New York: Guilford Press.

Widom, C. S. (1989). Does violence beget violence? A critical examination of the literature. *Psychological Bulletin, 106,* 3-28.

Williams-Peterson, M. G., Myers, B. J., Degen, M. H., Knisley, J. S., Elswick, R. K., & Schnoll, S. S. (1994). Drug-using and nonusing women: Potential for child abuse, child-rearing attitudes, social support, and affection for expected baby. *The International Journal of the Addictions, 29,* 1631-1643.

Windle, M. (1994). Substance use, risky behaviors, and victimization among a US national adolescent sample. *Addiction, 89,*175-182.

Wyatt, G. E., Guthrie, D., & Notgrass, C. M. (1992). Differential effects of women's child sexual abuse and subsequent sexual revictimization. *Journal of Consulting and Clinical Psychology, 60,* 167-173.

Zuravin, S., McMillen, C., DePanfilis, D., & Risley-Curtis, C. (1996). The intergenerational cycle of child maltreatment: Continuity versus discontinuity. *Journal of Interpersonal Violence, 11* (3), 315-334.

Racial Differences
in Neighborhood Disadvantage
Among Childbearing Women in New York City:
1991-1992

Kim D. Jaffee
Janet D. Perloff

SUMMARY. An ecological framework is utilized in this study to explore the differential neighborhood environments that existed for Black and White childbearing women in New York City during the early 1990s. We examined ecological risk factors for different racial groups in a highly segregated metropolitan city and provide a framework from which we can address issues of oppression and social inequality. This study examines neighborhood conditions and determines the extent to which Black and White women, who gave birth during 1991 and 1992, occupy differing neighborhoods in New York City and in each of the boroughs that comprise New York City–Manhattan, Bronx, Brooklyn, and Queens (excluding Staten Island).

Kim D. Jaffee, PhD, is Assistant Professor, College of Human Services and Health Professions, School of Social Work, Syracuse University, Syracuse, NY 13244 (E-mail: kdjaffee@syr.edu).

Janet D. Perloff, PhD, is Professor and Associate Dean for Research, School of Social Welfare, University at Albany, State University of New York, Albany, NY 12222 (E-mail: jperloff@uamail.albany.edu).

This project was supported by grant number R03 HS10061 from the Agency for Health Care Policy and Research.

[Haworth co-indexing entry note]: "Racial Differences in Neighborhood Disadvantage Among Childbearing Women in New York City: 1991-1992." Jaffee, Kim D., and Janet D. Perloff. Co-published simultaneously in *Journal of Human Behavior in the Social Environment* (The Haworth Social Work Practice Press, an imprint of The Haworth Press, Inc.) Vol. 7, No. 3/4, 2003, pp. 59-77; and: *Women and Girls in the Social Environment: Behavioral Perspectives* (ed: Nancy J. Smyth) The Haworth Social Work Practice Press, an imprint of The Haworth Press, Inc., 2003, pp. 59-77. Single or multiple copies of this article are available for a fee from The Haworth Document Delivery Service [1-800-HAWORTH, 9:00 a.m. - 5:00 p.m. (EST). E-mail address: docdelivery@haworthpress.com].

Digital Object Identifier: 10.1300/J137v7n03_05

High and persistent residential segregation of Blacks and Whites in NYC has put Black women at a clear and significant ecological disadvantage compared to White women regardless of the borough where they lived when they gave birth to their infant. This study found that, when compared to White women, Black women in New York City are at a vast disadvantage regardless of income. In Manhattan and Queens that disparity is the greatest with low income Black women much more likely than low income White women to live in a high poverty neighborhood. Overall, in NYC and across the four boroughs studied, low income Blacks were more likely than Whites to live in neighborhoods characterized by high poverty rates, substance abuse and inadequate health care. *[Article copies available for a fee from The Haworth Document Delivery Service: 1-800-HAWORTH. E-mail address: <docdelivery@haworthpress. com> Website: <http://www.HaworthPress.com> © 2003 by The Haworth Press, Inc. All rights reserved.]*

KEYWORDS. Race, ecological risk, residential segregation, women

INTRODUCTION

The profession of social work has long been committed to the creation of optimal social, physical and economic environments for all people. An ecological perspective allows for the study of the ongoing relationship between individuals and their environment (Germain, 1991). In many urban areas certain racial groups live in neighborhoods that produce demands and stressors that are difficult to overcome and create a sense of helplessness, despair and lowered self-esteem (Lazarus & Launier, 1978). These environments contain "social pollutions" such as poverty, structural unemployment, income inequality, and inadequate housing, education and health care. Destructive and disadvantaged communities that result from these social problems are the byproduct of institutional racism that manifests itself through policies, procedures and actions in housing markets that exclude certain groups from living where they choose.

The health and well-being of large numbers of minority women are jeopardized as these social disadvantages place "enormous adaptive burdens" on individuals and communities over time (Germain, 1991). Most studies examining racial and ethnic disparities in women's health focus on individual factors that place some women and their children at heightened risk for ill health. Social indicators that characterize the environment in which a woman resides have been previously neglected in health outcomes research.

An ecological framework is utilized in this study to explore the differential neighborhood environments that existed for Black and White childbearing women in New York City during the early 1990s. This perspective permits the examination of ecological risk factors for different racial groups in a highly segregated metropolitan city and provides a framework from which we can address issues of oppression and social inequality. This study will examine neighborhood conditions and determine the extent to which Black and White women, who gave birth during 1991 and 1992, occupy differing neighborhoods in New York City and in each of the boroughs which comprise New York City, Manhattan, Bronx, Brooklyn, and Queens (excluding Staten Island).

LITERATURE REVIEW

Residential Segregation

A number of previous studies have found a significant association between Black mortality rates and residential segregation (Collins & Williams, 1999; LaVeist, 1989; Polednak, 1996). The residential segregation of Blacks and Whites is a major facet of the urban landscape in the United States. Black/White ("Black" will refer to "Non-Hispanic Black" and "White" will refer to "Non-Hispanic White") segregation has remained quite high since 1970. The dissimilarity index is one of the indices of residential segregation and is used to measure the degree to which Blacks and Whites are segregated from one another. A score of 1.00 would indicate complete segregation and a score of .00 would indicate complete integration. In 1970 segregation indices in 29 large urban cities averaged about .83 (using the index of dissimilarity-D) indicating that 83 percent of Blacks would have to move from their neighborhoods to achieve an even residential pattern of Blacks and Whites in a given city (Massey, 1994). Many optimistically believed that the Civil Rights Act of 1968 banning racial discrimination in the sale and rental of housing would reduce residential segregation in cities over time. Sadly, twenty years later, in 1990, the residential segregation of Blacks and Whites in New York City remained extremely high (D = .83) (Frey & Farley, 1996; Massey & Denton, 1993).

An examination of racial segregation trends in New York City from 1970 to 1990 shows that Blacks and Whites are highly segregated in New York City (Jaffee, 1999; Massey & Denton, 1987). Two exposure indices were examined, one that measured the degree of Black interaction with Whites, and another that measured the degree of Black isolation from Whites. Lower interaction scores indicated a greater degree of residential segregation because the lower the score, the less likely it was that Blacks and Whites shared a common area (range from 1.00 to .00). Conversely, a high isolation score indicated greater residential segregation because it measures the degree to which Blacks encounter other Blacks in their neighborhood (range from 1.00 to .00). When this score is high it means that Blacks are living in relative isolation from Whites.

Racial segregation scores in New York City reveal a steady and significant decline in Black interaction with Whites between 1970 and 1990 in New York City. Furthermore, they also show an increase in Black isolation over the 20 year period. Black isolation increased from .59 in 1970 to .64 in 1990 (Jaffee, 1999; Massey & Denton, 1987). Overall, the likelihood of Blacks interacting with Whites in their neighborhood of residence was low and has declined substantially between 1970 and 1990 (from .21 to .11). These rather dismal trends indicate that as the proportion of Blacks increase they are becoming increasingly segregated from Whites in NYC.

There is a clear association between residential segregation, poverty, and other social and economic conditions at the metropolitan area level (Massey, Gross, & Eggers, 1991). We also know from previous research that high levels of segregation in cities confine poverty to spatially distinct neighborhoods where minority members tend to be clustered (Massey & Denton, 1988). As residential segregation increases, it is hypothesized that neighborhood poverty and disadvantage will also grow. In fact a New York City planning agency predicts that the population of the Bronx will be entirely Black and Hispanic by the early years of the next century, ". . . outside of a handful of de facto segregated enclaves of White people and a few essentially detached communities like Riverdale. By that time, the Bronx and Harlem and Washington Heights will make up a vast and virtually uninterrupted ghetto with a population close to that of Houston, Texas" (Kozol, 1995). This has enormous implications not only for the health of New York City residents, but for the health of residents of large northeast cities where segregation continues to increase.

Previous work by Polednak (1996) and LeVeist (1989, 1990) support the importance of political structure and economic forces on maternal and child health. This framework implies that discrimination and segregation perpetuate concentrated poverty for Blacks (LaVeist, 1989; Massey, 1994; Polednak, 1996). This concentration of high poverty for Blacks is associated with a whole host of neighborhood-level risk factors for poor maternal and child health such as infant mortality, low birthweight, maternal mortality, and childhood neglect and abuse[1] (Fossett & Perloff, 1999). Any structural process (such as residential segregation) that concentrates poverty will concentrate associated neighborhood risk factors as well (Massey & Denton, 1993). Therefore, these "concentration" effects may be important for explaining racial variation in social environments and consequent maternal and child health.

Neighborhood Risk

Concentrated poverty grew among Blacks between 1980 and 1990, and during this time period, the percentage of urban Blacks living in census tracts where 40 percent or more of the population was poor (high poverty area) increased from 20.2 percent to 23.7 percent. The percentage of poor urban Blacks who were living in these high poverty areas increased from 37.2 percent to 45.4 percent (Jargowsky, 1994, 1997). Those living in high poverty areas are disproportionately minority—more than 50 percent were non-Hispanic Black and 33 percent were Hispanic. Only 12 percent were White, even though Whites represent 75 percent of the U.S. population.

When individuals live in high poverty neighborhoods they encounter an "urban opportunity structure" that restricts socioeconomic mobility (Galster, 1996). These urban opportunity restrictions present themselves as "segregated housing, lack of positive role models as neighbors, limitations on capital, inferior public services, lower-quality public education, more violent/drug-infested neighborhoods, and impaired access to employment and job-related information networks" (Galster, 1996). Furthermore, in high poverty neighborhoods health care opportunities are severely limited. Poor minority neighborhoods not only fail to attract business and retail establishments, they also fail to attract medical practices because of neighborhood undesirability or the preponderance of non-lucrative Medicaid patients (Perloff, 1992; Perloff & Fossett, 1997; Perloff, Kletke, Fossett, & Banks, 1997). Communities with a high proportion of minorities have substantially lower ratios of health professionals than similar communities with primarily White residents (U.S. Department of Health and Human Services [DHHS], 1985). Not surprising, Blacks experience more difficulty accessing medical care than their White counterparts, particularly in high poverty neighborhoods (Blendon, Aiken, Freeman, & Corey, 1989).

Neighborhoods that experience high levels of social and economic disadvantage also have high rates of maternal mortality, infant mortality and low birthweight (Collins & David, 1990; Coulton & Pandey, 1992; Coulton, Pandey, & Chow, 1990; Roberts, 1997). One theoretical perspective presented by David and Collins (1991) is that racism, and consequently discrimination, are responsible for a large part of the Black-White differences observed in health outcomes. Therefore, racial differences in health outcomes come about through social and political mechanisms.

One common approach to the study of discrimination and health is to compare health outcomes of members of different racial/ethnic groups at the same socioeconomic level. Investigating whether adverse outcomes are equally likely among different groups at each socioeconomic level addresses the possible interaction between race and class. If differences persist after analyses that control for SES, then it can be assumed that race/ethnicity is independently associated with health status. One problem with this approach is that it assumes that environmental conditions are comparable within each SES category and that there is enough overlap in the two groups' SES distribution to permit adjusting for social class. Therefore, this research will seek to answer the following questions: Do Black and White women who gave birth in New York City live in significantly different environments? In each of the four New York City boroughs studied, what are the odds that a Black versus a White woman will live in a disadvantaged environment? When socioeconomic status is controlled, do Black and White women who gave birth occupy similar neighborhood environments?

METHODS

Data Sources

Utilizing 1991-1992 vital statistics birth records for New York City (NYC), the United Hospital Fund (UHF) NYC Community Health Atlas database (United Hospital Fund, 1994), and the 1990 U.S. Census data, we created a multi-level dataset that includes both individual and neighborhood-level variables (Perloff & Jaffee, 1997; Perloff & Jaffee, 1999). The NYC vital statistics birth records used in this study include all singleton live births to Black and White New York City (excluding

Staten Island) residents between January 1, 1991 and December 31, 1992. Any records that lacked the zip code necessary to link the neighborhood level variables to the woman's birth record were excluded (< 1%). The resulting dataset consisted of 138,761 Black and White women who were NYC residents and gave birth to a singleton infant in 1991 or 1992.

The UHF Zip Code Area Profiles (United Hospital Fund, 1994) contain information that describes a number of zip code characteristics in NYC. After an aggregation procedure for zip codes with less than 6,000 residents, 165 zip codes in NYC are represented, and these contain anywhere from 6,942 to 107,197 residents. This is a rich database in that it brings together numerous data sources, aggregated over a common geographic area.

Substance abuse hospital discharges rates, included in the UHF database, were used to measure neighborhood safety/quality, and ambulatory sensitive condition (ASC) hospitalization rates, also included in the UHF dataset, were used as an indicator of access to primary health care. High rates of substance abuse hospitalizations imply high rates of drug dealing and drug use which have been associated with crime and violence. Neighborhoods with these traits have been characterized as dangerous and unsafe for the majority of residents. High ASC hospitalization rates in a neighborhood are associated with barriers to accessing primary or ambulatory care. These barriers have been found to prevent individuals from getting the necessary primary care before their health condition reaches a point requiring hospitalization (Billings et al., 1993).

In addition, physician licensure data (also included in the UHF database) provided information on the supply of obstetricians and gynecologists for each zip code in New York City. The number of office and hospital-based physicians by specialty was obtained from the New York State Department of Education's Division of Professional Licensing Service's 1992 Physician Survey.

The Summary Tape File 3A (STF3A) from the U.S. Bureau of the Census was used to measure poverty level, per capita income, and the proportion of Blacks and Hispanics for each census tract in New York City.

Measures

Two individual-level variables were collected from the vital statistics birth record to describe the woman at the time she gave birth. The independent variable in this study is race and is measured as a dichotomous variable. Black women were coded as 1 and White women were coded as 0. The insurance status of the woman at the time she gave birth was used in the second part of the analysis as an indicator of socioeconomic status. Both Black and White women were considered low income if the birth of their infant was covered by Medicaid insurance or they were un-insured at the time of the birth. While this is a crude indicator of individual socioeconomic status, it is the only gauge of individual income available from the birth certificate.

There are a number of neighborhood-level dependent variables that will be examined in this analysis. The variables that measured economic and demographic characteristics of the woman's neighborhood were measured at the census tract level and extracted from the U.S. Census file. These variables were dichotomized in the following way. Those living in census tracts where: (1) 40% or more of the households live below poverty were coded as *high poverty*; (2) 60% or more of the residents are Black were coded as *high % Black*; (3) 60% or more of the residents are Hispanic were coded as *high % Hispanic;* (4) per capita income of less than $8000 was coded as *< $8000 per capita income.*

Neighborhood-level safety/quality and access to health care were measured at the zip code level and the dichotomous variables used to measure these factors include: (1) high substance abuse hospitalization rates among residents of the neighborhood measured as one standard deviation above NYC rate; (2) high ambulatory sensitive condition (ASC) hospitalization rates among residents measured as one standard deviation above the NYC rate; and (3) living in a obstetrician/gynecologists (ob/gyn) shortage area defined by using a guideline of 12 obstetrician/gynecologists per 100,000 population.[2] A previous study found that compared to primary care physicians overall, obstetricians and gynecologists are in considerably shorter supply in New York City's high poverty neighborhoods than in its low poverty neighborhoods (Perloff & Fossett, 1997). Each individual record will have these neighborhood level descriptors to characterize the neighborhood economic, safety, and health access risks of the woman when she gave birth.

Data Analysis

First, the association between race and neighborhood-level factors (such as economic indicators, racial/ethnic indicators, neighborhood quality indicators, and health care access indicators) is examined for women who gave birth during 1991-1992 in New York City. This is reported for New York City (excluding Staten Island) and each of the four boroughs by race.

Second, unadjusted odds ratios are presented for the neighborhood-level factors, showing the likelihood that Blacks versus Whites will live in disadvantaged neighborhoods. For example, is there a greater likelihood that a Black woman compared to a White woman who gave birth lived in an economically depressed neighborhood?

Finally, in an effort to control for individual economic differences between Black and White women in NYC and across the boroughs, we examine specifically whether *low income* Black and White women occupied similarly disadvantaged neighborhoods in each borough and NYC.

RESULTS

Neighborhood Risk Factors by Borough and Race

The association between race (Black and White), and neighborhood risk factors in New York City and in each of the boroughs (Manhattan, Bronx, Brooklyn, and Queens) are reported in Table 1. Additionally, a more precise way of examining the disparity in a Black woman versus a White woman's probability of living in a disadvantaged neighborhood was to look at the unadjusted odds ratios of the neighborhood-level factors for Black versus White women who gave birth in New York City and each of the boroughs (Table 2).

Overall in New York City there was a statistically significant association between race and each of the neighborhood economic, racial/ethnic, quality, and health care access indicators (Table 1). In fact, in NYC fewer than 10 percent of White women who gave birth possessed any one of the neighborhood risk factors, with the exception of living in an ob/gyn shortage area (Table 1).

Conversely, Black women who gave birth in NYC were much more likely to live in neighborhoods considered high risk. Over one-third of Black women (35.6%) lived in neighborhoods where per capita income was less than $8000, which was 4 times more likely for Black women than for White women. One-third (32.3%) of Black women who gave birth lived in high substance abuse neighborhoods, and another 18.1 percent lived in neighborhoods with high ambulatory sensitive condition hospitalizations compared to 5.6 percent and 1.8 percent, respectively, for White women.

TABLE 1. Neighborhood Characteristics of Childbearing Women by NYC Borough and Race: 1991-1992

VARIABLES	MANHATTAN		BRONX		BROOKLYN		QUEENS		TOTAL NYC	
	White	Black	White	Black	White	Black	White	Black	White	Black
	%	%	%	%	%	%	%	%	%	%
	N = 11,994	N = 9,448	N = 4,863	N = 17,396	N = 25,183	N = 35,860	N = 18,306	N = 15,711	N = 60,346	N = 78,415
NEIGHBORHOOD VARIABLES										
Economic Indicators										
High % Poverty	2.5	36.4	9.5	44.4	10.4	22.1	0.6	9.3	6.1	26.4
< $8000 Per Capita Income	3.4	45.6	14.6	56.8	14.2	33.2	1.1	10.3	8.5	35.6
Racial/Ethnic Indicators										
High % Black	1.2	55.2	2.3	22.1	4.0	77.2	1.6	61.4	2.6	59.4
High % Hispanic	4.1	13.7	9.8	25.5	3.2	3.8	1.4	0.9	3.4	9.3
Quality/Safety Indicator										
High Substance Abuse Rate	15.1	67.7	16.7	58.0	3.0	25.1	0	0	5.6	32.3
Health Care Access Indicators										
High ASC Rate	2.2	49.9	5.5	31.7	2.1	9.4	0.2	3.6	1.8	18.1
OB/GYN Shortage Area	20.9	66.2	74.2	82.0	62.9	68.5	80.3	84.5	60.7	74.4

All associations between race and neighborhood characteristics were statistically significant (X^2; $P < .0001$).

In terms of the magnitude of the Black/White disparity in neighborhood risk factors, overall in NYC Black women giving birth were 5.5 times more likely to live in a high poverty neighborhood than were their White counterparts (Table 2). Black women who gave birth in NYC were 8 times more likely to live in a poor quality neighborhood–that is, a neighborhood with a high rate of substance abuse hospitalizations–compared to White women. Furthermore, Blacks were 12 times more likely to live in a neighborhood where health care access was poor as indicated by a high ambulatory sensitive condition rate.

While a statistically significant association between race and the neighborhood risk factors also existed within each borough, there was considerable variation in the magnitude of the Black-White disparities across the boroughs (Table 2). This is evidenced in the dramatic differences in the likelihood of Black versus White women living in disadvantaged neighborhoods within each borough.

Manhattan: In Manhattan the disparity in neighborhood risk factors between Blacks and Whites was largest, indicating that at least for childbearing women, income inequality between Blacks and Whites was exceptionally large. For example, in Manhattan, one of the eco-

TABLE 2. Unadjusted Odds Ratio for Black Compared to White Childbearing Women Living in a Disadvantaged Neighborhood by NYC Borough: 1991-1992

VARIABLES	MANHATTAN		BRONX		BROOKLYN		QUEENS		TOTAL NYC	
	Odds Ratio	CI 95%	Odds Ratio	CI 95%	Odds Ratio	CI 95%	Odds Ratio	CI 95%	Odds Ratio	CI 95%
NEIGHBORHOOD VARIABLES										
Economic Indicators										
% High Poverty	21.9	(19.4, 24.8)	7.6	(6.9, 8.5)	2.5	(2.3, 2.6)	18.4	(14.6, 23.1)	5.5	(5.3, 5.8)
% < $8000 Per Capita Income	23.6	(21.2, 26.3)	7.7	(7.0, 8.4)	3.0	(2.9, 3.1)	10.6	(8.9, 12.5)	5.9	(5.7, 6.1)
Racial/Ethnic Indicators										
High % Black	102.7	(86.3, 122.2)	12.3	(9.9, 15.1)	81.7	(76.2, 87.5)	95.6	(83.5, 109.4)	53.9	(51.1, 57.0)
High % Hispanic	3.7	(3.3, 4.1)	3.1	(2.8, 3.5)	1.2	(1.1, 1.3)	0.6	(.5, .8)	2.9	(2.7, 3.0)
Quality/Safety Indicator										
High Substance Abuse Rate	11.8	(11.0, 12.6)	6.9	(6.3, 7.4)	11.0	(10.2, 11.9)	0	0	8.1	(7.8, 8.4)
Health Care Access Indicators										
High ASC Rate	43.5	(38.3, 49.4)	8.0	(7.1, 9.1)	5.0	(4.5, 5.5)	20.4	(14.4, 29.0)	12.0	(11.3, 12.8)
OB/GYN Shortage	7.4	(7.0, 7.9)	1.6	(1.5, 1.7)	1.3	(1.2, 1.3)	1.3	(1.3, 1.4)	1.9	(1.8, 1.9)

nomic indicators showed that only 3.4 percent of White women who gave birth during the study years lived in a very poor neighborhood (where per capita income was less than $8000) compared to almost half of Black woman (46%) (Table 2). A Black woman who gave birth in Manhattan was 22 times more likely than a White women who gave birth to live in a high poverty neighborhood (Table 2). The odds of a Black woman compared to a White woman living in a neighborhood in Manhattan with limited access to primary care was 43.5. Manhattan was the only borough where there was a significant association between race and living in an ob/gyn shortage area (health access indicator), with Black woman who gave birth over 7 times more likely to live in an ob/gyn shortage area than White women who gave birth.

Queens: Black women who gave birth in Queens were similar to Black women who gave birth in Manhattan in that they had a very high probability of living in a high poverty neighborhood when compared to White women (OR = 18.4). Living in a neighborhood with a high ambulatory sensitive condition rate was 20 times more likely among Black versus White women who gave birth in Queens.

Bronx: Disparities in neighborhood risks between Black and White women who gave birth in the Bronx were smaller than those found in Manhattan. In the Bronx Blacks were about 8 times more likely to live in a high poverty neighborhood than White women. Even though Black compared to White women who gave birth in the Bronx were at elevated risk for living in a high substance abuse (poor quality) neighborhood and a neighborhood with poor access to health care, the Black/White disparity was smaller in the Bronx for these risks than for New York City as a whole (Table 2).

Brooklyn: In Brooklyn the association between race and the neighborhood-level variables was weakest, with the exception of living in a high substance abuse neighborhood, where Black women were 11 times more likely to live in a high substance abuse neighborhood than Whites (Table 2). In Brooklyn the odds ratio for a Black woman compared to a White woman who gave birth and was living in a high poverty neighborhood was the smallest–only 2.5.

Neighborhood Conditions of Low-Income Women

It has been suggested that the geographic separation of Blacks and Whites may be attributed to different individual economic circumstances (Boger, 1996). Therefore, some assume that residential segregation is simply a result of Black and White income differences. To determine whether Black and White women of similar income levels live in comparable disadvantaged neighborhoods, we control for socioeconomic status by only considering low income Black and White women in this part of the analysis (N = 70,087).

Table 3 shows the proportion of low income White and Black women in the study who occupied neighborhoods that were significantly disadvantaged because of high poverty, high drug abuse hospitalization rates, and high ambulatory sensitive condition (ASC) hospitalization rates. If socioeconomic status is a strong determinant of where individuals live, regardless of race, we would expect that similar proportions of low income Black and White women would live in disadvantaged neighborhoods. To determine whether low income Blacks and low income Whites occupy similarly disadvantaged neighborhoods, we examined the bivariate relationship between race (Black vs. White), and neighborhood environment (high poverty vs. not high poverty; high substance abuse vs. not high substance abuse; and high ASC rate vs. not high ASC rate) for low income childbearing women in each borough (excluding Staten Island) and NYC.

For New York City overall, slightly more than two-thirds of Black women and one-third of White women were considered low income at the time they gave birth (Table 3). In NYC overall, almost 3 times as many low

TABLE 3. Neighborhood Characteristics of Low Income Childbearing Women by NYC Borough and Race: 1991-1992

VARIABLES	MANHATTAN		BRONX		BROOKLYN		QUEENS		TOTAL NYC	
	White %	Black %	White %	Black %	White %	Black %	White %	Black %	White %	Black %
Low Income Women	15.6	75.0	39.5	71.6	42.1	70.9	29.2	62.6	32.9	70.0
Low Income Women Living in High Poverty Neighborhood	10.3	39.1	19.2	51.0	15.0	25.8	1.5	12.2	11.8	31.0
Low Income Women Living in High Substance Abuse Neighborhood	25.0	70.1	36.6	65.5	3.9	27.3	0.0	0.0	8.1	37.0
Low Income Women Living in High ASC Hosp. Neighborhood	8.6	51.1	12.7	37.0	4.1	10.6	0.4	4.4	4.4	20.9

income Black women compared to White women who gave birth lived in economically depressed neighborhoods (31% and 11.8%, respectively). Furthermore, over one-third (37%) of low income Black women lived in a high substance abuse neighborhood, while only 8.1 percent of low income White women resided in such a neighborhood. Low income Black women were almost 5 times more likely to reside in a neighborhood where access to health care was low (a high ambulatory sensitive condition rate) compared to low income White women (Table 3).

Queens has the lowest proportion of low income Black women living in high poverty neighborhoods compared to the other boroughs; however, low income Blacks were 8 times more likely to live in a high poverty neighborhood compared to low income Whites within the borough of Queens. The disparity in the economic neighborhood risks among low income Blacks versus Whites giving birth is highest in Queens (12.2% vs. 1.5%), followed by Manhattan (39.1% vs. 10.3%), the Bronx (51.0% vs.19.2%), and Brooklyn (25.8% vs. 15.0%).

The highest proportion of low income Black women living in a high substance abuse neighborhood was in Manhattan, where a full 70% of low income Black women lived in such a neighborhood compared to 25% among low income White women. In terms of neighborhood access to health care, half of low income Black women in Manhattan were living in a neighborhood where residents experienced a high rate of hospitalizations for ambulatory sensitive conditions (ASC). The Bronx had the second highest proportion of low income Blacks living in high ASC neighborhoods (37.0%).

Manhattan and the Bronx had the largest proportion of low income Black women who lived in a high substance abuse neighborhood (70% and 65%, respectively). Queens had the lowest proportion of Blacks who lived in a high ASC neighborhood, yet had the greatest disparity between low income Blacks and Whites–low income Blacks were 11 times more likely to live in a high ASC neighborhood compared to low income Whites (4.4 vs. 0.4).

DISCUSSION

There is a clear and significant association between race and the neighborhood risk factors in New York City (excluding Staten Island) and the four NYC boroughs. Black women were significantly more likely than Whites to be at risk for living in a very disadvantaged neighborhood. There were large differences (across the boroughs) in the proportion of Black women who lived in economically depressed, poor quality neighborhoods where access to health care was lacking. In borough by borough comparisons, Black women who lived in Manhattan and the Bronx when they gave birth were much more likely than Black women in Brooklyn and Queens to live in a disadvantaged neighborhood. The patterns of neighborhood disadvantage observed in Manhattan and the Bronx are a stark result of the hypersegregation of Blacks and Whites in New York City as a whole (Jaffee, 1999). This study found that Manhattan and Queens had the highest probability that a Black woman versus a White woman would live in a disadvantaged neighborhood. Whites in Manhattan and Queens were relatively advantaged compared to those in Brooklyn and the Bronx. Consequently, the disparity in neighborhood disadvantage between Blacks and Whites was highest in Manhattan and Queens. Also, the odds of a Black versus a White woman living in a neighborhood that was primarily Black (60% or more Black) was highest in Manhattan and Queens. Even though Blacks in Queens were much less likely than Blacks in other boroughs to live in high risk neighborhoods, the income disparities between Blacks and Whites within Queens were as large as those found in Manhattan. The low proportion of Blacks who lived in disadvantaged neighborhoods in Queens was a result of the small number of disadvantaged neighborhoods that exist in Queens. However, Blacks are much more likely than Whites to live in those neighborhoods. Residential segregation makes it more likely that Blacks versus Whites will live in disadvantaged neighborhoods.

Income disparities between Blacks and Whites in Brooklyn were small relative to the other boroughs. In Brooklyn, White women were more likely to live in a high poverty neighborhood in comparison to White women in the other boroughs. Alternately, Blacks in Brooklyn were less likely to live in high poverty neighborhoods compared to Blacks in the Bronx and Manhattan. The disparities in neighborhood risk for Blacks and Whites in Manhattan and Queens were quite high compared to Brooklyn and the Bronx. Income inequality appears to be most evident in Manhattan and Queens.

Clearly, when compared to White women, Black women in New York City are at a vast disadvantage regardless of income. In Queens that disparity is the greatest, with low income Black women 8 times more likely than low income White women to live in a high poverty neighborhood. Overall, in NYC and across the four boroughs studied, low income Blacks were more likely than low income Whites to live in neighborhoods characterized by high poverty rates, substance abuse and inadequate health care.

High and persistent residential segregation of Blacks and Whites in NYC has put Black women at a clear and significant ecological disadvantage compared to White women regardless of the borough where they lived when they gave birth to their infant. Spatially, Manhattan and the Bronx contain large contiguous high poverty areas inhabited by a large proportion of minority residents. Brooklyn and Queens had a smaller proportion of Black women who lived in neighborhoods characterized by economic depression and poor access to health care. However, in Queens the high Black/White disparity in the neighborhood risk factors suggests Black women are much more likely to be relegated to disadvantaged neighborhoods than their White counterparts.

Although this study was able to use readily available neighborhood data, the indicator for neighborhood quality/safety (substance abuse hospitalization rates) was somewhat crude. There are a variety of ways that researchers measure neighborhood, and while zip code is probably adequate as a general measure of social and economic conditions, smaller spatial units such as block groups have been identified as more appropriate for the study of neighborhood risk.

IMPLICATIONS

The Healthy People 2010 objectives articulate specific goals to eliminate maternal and child health disparities between racial and ethnic minority groups by the year 2010. As part of the Initiative to Eliminate Disparities in Health, the federal government has reinforced the principle of equity by moving the nation from the goal of *reducing* disparities to one of *eliminating* disparities in health (U.S. Department of Health and Human Services, [DHHS],1999). The findings from this study support prior research showing that Whites live in neighborhoods that are qualitatively better than those of Blacks (Wilson, 1987). These superior living conditions are protective for White women's health, while disadvantaged living conditions among Black women present a multitude of health risks. This study also lends support to ecological studies that have shown that SES among poor Black compared to poor White households is not equivalent (Krivo & Peterson, 1996). Poor Blacks continue to live in neighborhoods that are qualitatively different than poor Whites. An investment in improved living conditions for Black women in segregated inner cities will go a long way toward eliminating health disparities.

Historically, social workers provided a holistic, ecological approach to serving ill clients. This is accomplished by not only assessing a client's physical and psychosocial needs, but environmental health needs as well (Dhooper, 1997). The multi-dimensional quality of social worker responsibilities in maternal and child health settings provides opportunities for those in the social work profession to target not only individual risk factors associated with poor health but to simultaneously target larger social determinants of racial health disparities through advocacy and social change. Social workers can use existing research and available data to engage policymakers and government representatives in developing policies that will help increase low-income women's access to primary care (Gaston, Barrett, Johnson, & Epstein, 1998).

If health is intimately tied to social and environmental conditions, then it behooves us to focus a significant portion of intervention at the community and policy levels rather than at the level of the individual client (Minkler, Wallace, & McDonald, 1994). Social workers have an important contribution to make toward achieving the important national social justice goal of equalizing health status and access for all (Gaston et al., 1998). Furthermore, even though developing public health intervention programs and increased access to medical care are fruitful goals to improve maternal and child health in poor neighborhoods, they can be seen as only partial solutions to problems which are reflective of deeper societal ills. The racial separation of Blacks is a result of entrenched institutional and individual racism. If segregation of Blacks from Whites continues, poverty will expand and persist in our nation's cities, as will the health disparities between Blacks and Whites. If we hope to close the gap between Black and White health outcomes, we must confront the many forms of racism that pervade our society.

NOTES

1. High levels of drug use and violence that occur in high poverty neighborhoods increase the likelihood of child neglect and maltreatment. Parents living in high poverty neighborhoods were five times more likely to maltreat their children than those living in higher income neighborhoods (Olds, 1988; Sedlack, 1989).

2. These guidelines were developed by the Capacity Building Subcommittee of the New York State Medicaid Managed Care Advisory Committee (New York State, 1995, August).

REFERENCES

Billings, J., Zeitel, L., Lukomnik, J., Carey, T. S., Blank, A. E., & Newman, L. (1993). Impact of socioeconomic status on health care use in New York City. *Health Affairs, 12*(1), 162-173.

Blendon, R. J., Aiken, L. H., Freeman, H. E., & Corey, C. R. (1989). Access to medical care for Black and White Americans. A matter of continuing concern. *Journal of the American Medical Association, 261*(2), 278-281.

Boger, C. J. (1996). Toward ending residential segregation: A fair share proposal for the next reconstruction. In J. C. Boger & J. W. Wegner (Eds.), *Race, poverty, and American cities*. Chapel Hill, N.C.: University of North Carolina Press.

Collins, C. A., & Williams, D. R. (1999). Segregation and mortality: The deadly effect of racism. *Sociological Forum, 14*(3), 495-523.

Collins, J. W., & David, R. J. (1990). The differential effect of traditional risk factors on infant birthweight among Blacks and Whites in Chicago. *American Journal of Public Health, 80*(6), 679-682.

Coulton, C., & Pandey, S. (1992). Geographic concentration of poverty and risk to children in urban neighborhoods. *American Behavioral Scientist, 35*, 238-257.

Coulton, C., Pandey, S., & Chow, J. (1990). Concentration of poverty and the changing ecology of low-income urban neighborhoods: An analysis of the Cleveland area. *Social Work Research and Abstracts, 26*, 5-16.

David, R. J., & Collins, J. W. (1991, Summer). Bad outcomes in Black babies: Race or racism. *Ethnicity and Disease, 1*, 236-244.

Dhooper, S. (1997). *Social work in health care in the 21st century*. Thousand Oaks, California: Sage Publications.

Fossett, J. W., & Perloff, J. D. (1999). The "new" health reform and access to care: The problem of the inner city. In D. Rowland, S. Rosenbaum, A. Salganicoff, & M. Lillie-Blanton (Eds.), *Access to health care: Promises and prospects for low income Americans*. Washington, D.C.: Kaiser Commission on Medicaid and the Uninsured.

Frey, W. H., & Farley, R. (1996). Latino, Asian, and Black Segregation in U.S. Metropolitan Areas: Are Multiethnic Metros Different? *Demography, 33* (February), 35-50.

Galster, G. (1996). Polarization, place, and race. In J. C. Boger & J. W. Wegner (Eds.), *Race, poverty, and American cities.* Chapel Hill, North Carolina: The University of North Carolina Press.

Gaston, M. H., Barrett, S. E., Johnson, T. L., & Epstein, L. G. (1998). Health care needs of medically underserved women of color: The role of the Bureau of Primary Health Care. *Health and Social Work, 23*(2), 86-95.

Germain, C. B. (1991). *Human Behavior in the Social Environment.* New York, New York: Columbia University Press.

Jaffee, K. D. (1999). *An Ecological Analysis of Low Birthweight in New York City: The Role of Residential Segregation.* Unpublished Dissertation, SUNY at Albany, Albany, New York.

Jargowsky, P. (1994). Ghetto poverty among Blacks in the 1980's. *Journal of Policy Analysis and Management, 13*(2), 288-310.

Jargowsky, P. (1997). *Poverty and place: Ghettos, barrios, and the American city.* New York, New York: Russell Sage Foundation.

Kozol, J. (1995). *Amazing grace: The lives of children and the conscience of a nation.* New York, New York: Crown Publishers, Inc.

Krivo, L. J., & Peterson, R. D. (1996). Extremely disadvantaged neighborhoods and urban crime. *Social Forces, 75,* 619-648.

LaVeist, T. A. (1989). Linking residential segregation to the infant mortality race disparity in U.S. cities. *Sociology and Social Research, 73,* 90-94.

LaVeist, T. A. (1990). Simulating the effects of poverty on the race disparity in postneonatal mortality. *Journal of Public Health Policy,* 11(4), 463-73.

Lazarus, R. S., & Launier, R. (1978). *Stress-related transactions between person and environment.* New York, New York: Plenum.

Massey, D. S. (1994). America's Apartheid and the Urban Underclass. *Social Service Review* (December), 471-487.

Massey, D., & Denton, N. (1987). Trends in the residential segregation of Blacks, Hispanics, and Asians: 1970-1980. *American Sociological Review, 52* (December), 802-825.

Massey, D., & Denton, N. (1993). *American Apartheid: Segregation and the Making of the Underclass.* Cambridge, Massachusetts: Harvard University Press.

Massey, D., & Denton, N. (1988). The dimensions of residential segregation. *Social Forces, 67:2* (December), 281-313.

Massey, D. S., Gross, A. B., & Eggers, M. L. (1991). Segregation, the concentration of poverty, and the life chances of individuals. *Social Science Research, 20,* 397-420.

Minkler, M., Wallace, S. P., & McDonald, M. (1994). The political economy of health: A useful theoretical tool for health education practice. *International Quarterly of Community Health Education, 15*(92), 111-125.

New York State, Capacity Building Subcommittee. (1995, August). *Report to the Medicaid Managed Care Advisory Committee.*

Olds, D. (1988). The prenatal/early infancy project. In R. Price, E. Cowen, R. Lorian, & J. Ramos-Mckay (Eds.), *Ounces of prevention*. Washington, D.C.: American Psychological Association.

Perloff, J. (1992). Health care resources for children and pregnant women. *Journal of the Future of Children, 2*, 78-94.

Perloff, J., & Fossett, J. (1997). *Staffing Medicaid Managed Care: Physician supply and network capacity in New York City*: David and Lucile Packard Foundation.

Perloff, J., & Jaffee, K. (1997). Prenatal care utilization in New York City: Comparison of measures and assessment of their significance for urban health. *Bulletin of the New York Academy of Medicine, 74*(1), 51-64.

Perloff, J., & Jaffee, K. (1999). Late entry in prenatal care: The neighborhood context. *Social Work, 44*(3), 116-128.

Perloff, J. D., Kletke, P. R., Fossett, J. W., & Banks, S. (1997). Medicaid participation among urban primary care physicians. *Medical Care, 35*(2), 142-157.

Polednak, A. P. (1996). Trends in US urban Black infant mortality, by degree of residential segregation. *American Journal of Public Health, 86*(May), 723-726.

Polednak, A. P. (1997). *Segregation, poverty, and mortality in urban African Americans*. New York, New York: Oxford University Press.

Roberts, E. (1997). Neighborhood social environment and the distribution of low birthweight in Chicago. *American Journal of Public Health, 87*(4).

Sedlack, A. (1989). *National incidence of child abuse and neglect*. Paper presented at the biennial meeting of the Society for Research in Child Development, Kansas City.

United Hospital Fund. (1994). *The New York City Community Health Atlas*. New York: United Hospital Fund.

U. S. Department of Health and Human Services. (1985, August). *Report of the Secretary's Task Force on Black and Minority Health: Volume I*. Rockville, MD: Office of Minority Health.

U. S. Department of Health and Human Services. (1999). *Health People 2010: Health objectives for the nation*. Rockville, MD.

Wilson, W. J. (1987). *The truly disadvantaged: The inner city, the underclass, and public policy*. Chicago, Illinois: University of Chicago Press.

A Feminist Approach to Exploring the Intersections of Individuals, Families, and Communities: An Illustration Focusing on Lesbian Mother Research

Lucy R. Mercier
Rena D. Harold

SUMMARY. It is important for social workers to use contextual understandings to guide their work with client systems, particularly those whose life experiences fall under the umbrella of diversity. Thus, integrating women's perspectives/voices directly into the study of their lives is one way to more accurately understand lesbians, whose experiences as women, as partners, and as mothers may be misinterpreted without their own perspectives to guide understanding. This paper presents a model for research that utilizes an eco-systemic perspective, including eco maps and genograms, to collect and organize data. This model is a natu-

Lucy R. Mercier is affiliated with Saginaw Valley State University.

Rena D. Harold is affiliated with Michigan State University.

Address correspondence to: Lucy R. Mercier, Saginaw Valley State University Department of Social Work, 7400 Bay Road, University Center, MI 48710 (E-mail: amercier@svsu.edu).

[Haworth co-indexing entry note]: "A Feminist Approach to Exploring the Intersections of Individuals, Families, and Communities: An Illustration Focusing on Lesbian Mother Research." Mercier, Lucy R., and Rena D. Harold. Co-published simultaneously in *Journal of Human Behavior in the Social Environment* (The Haworth Social Work Practice Press, an imprint of The Haworth Press, Inc.) Vol. 7, No. 3/4, 2003, pp. 79-95; and: *Women and Girls in the Social Environment: Behavioral Perspectives* (ed: Nancy J. Smyth) The Haworth Social Work Practice Press, an imprint of The Haworth Press, Inc., 2003, pp. 79-95. Single or multiple copies of this article are available for a fee from The Haworth Document Delivery Service [1-800-HAWORTH, 9:00 a.m. - 5:00 p.m. (EST). E-mail address: docdelivery@haworthpress.com].

ral extension of social work interview and assessment techniques, and can illuminate respondents' diverse experiences as well as the socio-cultural environments in which these experiences are embedded. *[Article copies available for a fee from The Haworth Document Delivery Service: 1-800-HAWORTH. E-mail address: <docdelivery@haworthpress.com> Website: <http://www.HaworthPress.com>* © *2003 by The Haworth Press, Inc. All rights reserved.]*

KEYWORDS. Feminism, research methods, lesbian, eco maps

Traditional social science research has been criticized for ignoring women's experiences, misinterpreting women's responses, or dismissing women's issues as unimportant (Stacey & Thorne, 1985). Even when women's concerns have been addressed in research and practice, the limitations of conventional social science methods have impaired researchers' chances of producing results that are relevant for many women (Harding, 1991). Similarly, in the unique circumstances under which social scientists adequately address issues of gender, frameworks for knowledge often have failed to account for variance in women's experience in terms of ethnicity, sexual orientation, age and other axes of difference (Smith, 1990). These epistemological shortcomings limit the usefulness of conventional research. More importantly, restrictive frameworks for knowledge produce a climate of false knowledge, leading practitioners and researchers alike to accept as true the unproved assumptions upon which conventional social research is often based.

Feminist research is grounded in "an understanding that many aspects of women's experience have not yet been articulated or conceptualized within social science" (Jayaratne & Stewart, 1991, p. 89). Many contemporary feminist researchers also understand that "truth" or "knowledge" is subjectively related to the perspectives of the parties involved in the research interaction. In the case of lesbians, this re-conceptualization of knowledge building is particularly important, since lesbians continue to be largely marginalized by the dominant culture and by the practices of mainstream science. To better understand the experience of these women as they negotiate their social environments, additional research is needed that focuses on lesbian mother families and their communities.

A major theme of contemporary family research is its increasing recognition of diverse families (Berardo, 1991). As definitions of family move away from conventional gender constraints, new knowledge emerges that emphasizes an understanding of family as a complex and changeable arena for working through interpersonal, economic, political, and other relations (Ferree, 1991). Research on lesbian mothers is important because of its relationship to issues as diverse as gender roles in family life, understanding of family structure and function, the impact of social support and social policy on family life, and the role of individual experience in the success of families. Lesbian mother families "provide a fertile testing ground for family theories and simultaneously pose . . . challenges for dominant family theories" (Demo & Allen, 1996, p. 423).

One way to more accurately understand lesbians, whose experiences as women, as partners, and as mothers may be overlooked, misunderstood, or misinterpreted without their own perspectives to guide understanding, is to use research methods that integrate women's perspectives/voices directly into the study of their lives. Qualitative analysis is particularly useful for exploration of conditions and experiences that are not easily accessed by conventional, quantitative research methods. This approach is especially valuable in studying linkages between individuals, families, and communities because it takes a comprehensive and holistic perspective toward respondents' experiences. In this way, data collection can highlight respondents' experiences as well as the socio-cultural environments in which these experiences are embedded. In addition, utilizing an eco-systemic perspective to collect and organize data is a natural extension of social work interview and assessment techniques, making this model easily translatable for social work practitioners and researchers (Harold, Mercier, & Colarossi, 1997).

This paper describes a study in which feminist, qualitative analysis offered an opportunity to "give voice" to lesbians. This approach for conducting research interviews presents an opportunity for important advancements in understanding the complexity and variability of individual/family/community relationships in the lives of lesbian mothers. Although the study of such complex relationships can be unwieldy, it can produce rich results that enhance the understanding of social work researchers, practitioners, and policy makers. The methodology presented here as a tool for organizing in-depth research on the socio-cultural conditions of lesbian mother families is also applicable to other groups of women who are uniquely placed in history and social condition.

THE STUDY

A study was undertaken of lesbian mother families in an area of the Midwestern United States. This research project was a systematic, in-depth exploration of lesbian mothers' relationships within their households and between their households and the organizations and institutions around them. The rationale for the study was that lesbians are challenged by historical, structural, cultural, and interpersonal factors and that these conditions influence their experiences as members of families. Rather than focusing on problems, however, this study was designed to yield data that reflect both obstacles and opportunities for support in the respondents' familial and social interactions. Throughout the study, data collection focused on current interactions, the impact of noteworthy events in the past, and perceptions of everyday or routine exchanges within lesbian mother families and between families and their social environments.

Lesbian mothers were recruited for the study through questionnaires distributed in the women's community via many channels, including word-of-mouth, direct mailing to lesbian community centers, feminist bookstores, support groups and religious organizations, and distribution at social, educational, sporting, and political events. The questionnaire gathered demographic data about the individual respondent and her family and offered lesbian mothers the opportunity to volunteer for face-to-face interviews.

Over 150 women completed questionnaires and, of these, approximately 80% agreed to be interviewed. This paper describes the foundation for the process used to collect narratives from a subsample of 21 lesbian mothers. An overview of the study, including theoretical foundations and the interview methodology, are described below. These provide the background for a discussion of the use of qualitative interviewing for understanding human behavior in the social environment, particularly with oppressed populations.

ECO MAPS AND INTERVIEWS

Traditional methods of measuring family functioning rely heavily on standardized, quantitative measures and statistical analyses. When such methods are paired with rigorous sampling techniques, they are thought to produce conclusions that are generalizeable outside of the actual respondent base. One issue with such research is that it may not provide for a true, clear, or comprehensive picture of the experiences of the research respondents. In addition, data that are "crunched" in this way generally require a great deal of interpretation before they are comprehensible to consumers of information. Thus, the conventional system may privilege the researcher with designing the study; choosing and restricting the parameters of data collection; separating the information from the context in which it has most meaning; aggregating it; performing statistical tests on it; and then interpreting its meaning.

To center research on the intersections of individual, family and community experiences, a model is needed that emphasizes the impact of socio-cultural forces on the experiences of individuals and groups, and that privileges the context in which interactions occur (Bronfenbrenner, 1979; Germain, 1981). This perspective, commonly referred to as the eco-system model, is particularly appropriate for research that focuses on social justice for oppressed populations because it takes into account historical and geographical location, personal history and family of origin, biological and psychological factors, and a number of other conditions in attempting to understand the circumstances of people.

The eco-system model is sometimes conceptualized as a series of concentric circles with the individual at the center. Family, culture, environmental-structural factors, and historical contexts encase the individual, and each is considered as it intersects with the individual, and with each of the other factors. Researchers and practitioners who use the model contend that examination of the intersections between individuals and their social environments is useful because that is where conflict, oppression, and support occurs. For the purpose of examining the life experiences of lesbian mothers, the use of this model highlighted how interactions with members of their households, neighborhoods, schools, work places, and other systems impact their lives. Of course, interventions to restore health to individuals and institutions must take place in these intersections as well, making the model especially relevant for social workers and their search for ways to translate research into direct service and social action.

In searching for a way to collect and organize information that accounted for the complex eco-systems of the respondents, this project used a tool from the social work canon–the eco map (Hartman, 1978). [In an earlier study with heterosexual parent families, eco maps were also introduced into interviews as a way to stimulate discussion about the respondents' experiences with their families and communities (Harold et al., 1997).] Although eco maps are most commonly used as assessment tools in clinical settings, in this study, they were used to capture the socio-cultural context of the respondents' lives and to provide structure and focus for data collection interviews.

An eco map is a two-dimensional template for graphically representing relationships within a family and between a family and its social environment (Figure 1). In the interviews, each respondent completed an eco map by selecting and drawing a series of lines chosen from a key printed on the template while verbally describing the relationship in her own words. The lines, which depicted the primary characteristics of the interactions in the respondents' relationships, represented relationship types experienced by the woman.

Each interview started with the researcher and respondent drawing a genogram of the respondent's family in the "household" circle on the eco map. A genogram is a graphic representation of a family where individuals are represented by geometric figures such as circles or triangles (Carter & McGoldrick, 1980; McGoldrick & Gerson, 1985). Once the genogram was drawn, the participant selected lines to connect each member of the household with all other members.

For the remainder of the eco map, each respondent depicted relationships between her household and each system in her social environment by choosing and drawing in lines. Some respondents did not have relationships with every type of system printed on the eco map, and so did not indicate line types for those systems. Similarly, some respondents

FIGURE 1. Family eco map.

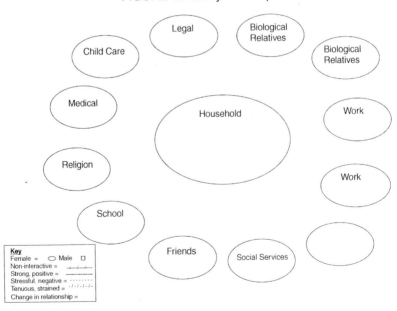

added systems to the eco map and so indicated additional lines. Each eco map, then, yielded a concise summary of perceived relationships within and around the respondent's family.

In addition to simplified measures of relationship type, in-depth information about the respondents' relationships was explored. As women selected and drew lines onto the eco maps, they began to talk about the ways in which they experienced their relationships. Verbal data from the interviews were documented directly onto the eco maps, as well as by the interviewer's notes and audio tape recordings. Notes written on the eco maps focused on themes articulated by the respondents, examples of stress or support in the environment, and rich descriptions of relationships within and around the families. These included content summaries, verbatim recording of statements, notes on non-verbal communication, and key words or phrases used during the interviews. These notes were checked with and verified by the respondents during the interviews, and in one instance, by telephone after the interview.

This strategy for collecting and organizing information proved to be surprisingly efficient. On average, in a two hour interview, an interviewer was able to collect, roughly organize, and verify information about the perceived strengths and weaknesses of the couple relationship (in two-parent homes), the respondent's and partner's (when present) relationships with each child, sibling relationships, and the relationships between the lesbian mother family and the work place, social services, mother's friends, children's school and child care, religious institutions, health care providers, the legal system, families of origin, and other relevant systems.

Although the eco map interviews were relatively structured, they were not rigid. The nature of the methodology used in this study allowed data collection to be a dynamic process for the interviewers and the respondents. The eco map guided each interview and acted as a non-verbal reminder of the study's primary focus on the respondents' relationships. Nevertheless, it also allowed for the introduction of many other topics and issues important to the respondents. For example, many participants provided historical data, particularly about coming out as lesbian and about the history of their partner relationship, which were peripherally related to the study (and important to our understanding of the context of their lives), but not directly covered on the eco map. This flexibility in methodology conformed to feminist research methods that privilege interviewees' determinations of relevant material and emphasize respondents' guidance of the research process (Reinharz, 1992). It also reflected the researchers' desire to integrate meaningful themes from all areas of the respondents' lives into the data in order to increase the potential for meaningful analyses.

ORGANIZING THE WOMEN'S VOICES

In planning for analysis of the interview data, the emphasis was on retaining the richness of the data gathered, preserving the unique quality of each interview, and emphasizing the context in which each story occurred. In doing so, the data analysis contributes toward an enhanced understanding of women in the social world, and suggests ways to move from understanding to planning for social change as an integral part of the feminist research process (Jayaratne & Stewart, 1991).

The fundamental plan for analyzing the narrative data in this study replicated a process developed in a similar study with heterosexual-parent families (Harold, Palmiter, Lynch, Freedman-Doan, & Eccles, 2000). This process utilized an interactive model of analysis, in which deductive and inductive approaches to analysis work together to produce richly detailed descriptive data, as well as new concepts and hypotheses (Strauss & Corbin, 1990). Initially, each completed eco map was viewed as a graphic representation of the level of support or stress experienced by the respondent and her family. That is, an eco map with many relationships described as "strong/positive" was seen as very different from an eco map with many "tenuous/strained" or "stressful/negative" relationships.

Although this picture of each woman's relationships was helpful in understanding her life, the interactions within the family, and between the family and outside systems, was of critical importance. To examine these interactions, the rich narrative data from the interviews were used to consider the relationships in greater detail. Interview data were coded into classifications determined by the major divisions on the eco maps (e.g., relationships between respondents and their partners, or relationships between households and school systems). Then, categories were derived from the content of the material within each classification. The categories were based on the comments of the respondents themselves, as well as on issues suggested by previous research with mothers and with lesbians. Finally, themes within categories were identified by examining the meanings of interviewee's responses.

For example, for each interview, all comments related to relationships within the household circle were coded into the family classification. Categories within the family classification included the relationship between the respondent and her partner, the relationships between parents and children, and the relationships between children in the household. Each of these categories contained several themes. To illustrate, two of the themes of the relationship between partnered lesbian mothers were: the centrality of the partner relationship; and the perceived importance of couple's complementary characteristics.

The considerable effort needed to sort and code data in this way was worthwhile because the analysis retained the richness of the women's experiences and reflected the unique circumstances of each family. Once data were organized by theme, the researchers were able to examine the experiences and perspectives of lesbian mothers from several different approaches. One way to analyze the data was to look across interviews at the similarities and differences found in the entire sample of lesbian mothers without losing the uniqueness of any woman. For example, Lisa[1], 24, who lives with her partner of 18 months and their 4-year-old daughter, described her partnership:

> (This is) a really good relationship . . . we support each other . . . (this is) a more equal power balance than any other relationship I've been in.

Cara, 46, who is a non-biological mother of a 6-month-old boy, also commented on the intensity of her relationship with her partner of 10 years, but with a different slant:

> I feel like we have a pretty honest . . . you know, in our relationship we pretty much tell each other everything pertinent. We don't have secrets from each other and, you know, I think that we think of each other as being really good friends. And I think that that's one of the reasons that this kind of relationship can work. That people of the same gender, especially women . . . because you can be friends before you're lovers if you take the time to develop the friendship, and it makes your relationship stronger.

Compare these with Candace's description of her two-year relationship with her partner:

> Our feelings for each other are so strong that it's almost like we think the same, we feel the same, . . . we cherish our relationship. It's like knowing that I'm always there for her and she's always there for me. (We are good at) making decisions, and, um, support-

ing each other just . . . kind of like confiding in each other. We're very good at that and we're best friends.

Each of these respondents focused on a different aspect of the partner relationship–equality, honesty, availability–but all emphasized the centrality of the couple relationship. In addition, these brief examples hint at the diverse personalities and perspectives of the women interviewed.

A second approach to examining the data was to look at responses to specific themes within families. That is, in families where two lesbian mothers were interviewed, this methodology allowed researchers to compare responses to intra-family and household-family interactions across couples. For example, Sheila and Marla, a couple with four small children, discussed the impact on their family of social attitudes toward lesbians. Although both identified anti-lesbian sentiment as a noxious social condition, their different approaches to the problem also reflected the characteristics of their interactions with the environment. Sheila is a teacher, and describes herself having limited control over her workplace environment. She framed the issue of social rejection in terms of its impact on behaviors and relationships primarily within her family:

> I think probably the thing that I notice the most is that we're probably not as affectionate or demonstrative with one another as we could be. And I think probably because we've grown so used to . . . you know . . . in 95% of . . . our lives (we are) not . . . able to really be demonstrative. And it's just kind of been a carry over, and we haven't made a huge effort to make sure that we continue to do that. I mean, it's not like we're void of that, and it's not like the kids never see us, you know, be affectionate with one another, but it's probably not as much as I would like them to see us.

In contrast, Marla is self-employed and, thus, more able to control social contact with disapproving others. Interestingly, Marla focused on attitudes toward lesbian and gay issues in Sheila's work place as a way to describe the importance of social approval and support.

> This work environment is so much better for her than her last work environment, where there was a principal who, just right in front of the whole school, was cutting down gays and everything. It was just the most awful environment. She was the only, that she *knew of*, gay person on the staff. Now this is a much different working

environment. She has open gay staff members and it feels much more supportive.

As these brief excerpts illustrate, analyzing data from all informants within families allows for examination of the ways in which similar circumstances and experiences are filtered through social role and position, geography, history, and individual character. In the study described here, examination of this type allowed the researchers to gain a full perspective of the remarkably consistent ways in which these women expressed their commitment to each other and their children, approached obstacles with creativity, and acted as advocates within their communities. At the same time, this approach allowed for explicit understanding of how individual respondents perceived and reacted to particular people and events in their social environments.

In addition to being able to look at themes across respondents, this methodology allowed an examination of themes within individual narratives. For example, Chandra, 32, told a highly emotional story about her ex-husband's attempts to gain sole custody of her children by asserting that her sexual orientation impaired her ability to parent. Chandra verbalized both doubt and anxiety that his case would win in court. If her statements about the custody case are studied in isolation from the remainder of her story, she appears to be overwhelmed and frozen with grief and anger, but thematic analysis across all classifications of relationships on the eco map reveals her as a woman with significant coping strategies. For example, in reference to her relationship with her daughter's school, Chandra noted that her child's ability to be open about her family was a sign of a healthy child, as well as a supportive school environment:

> (My six-year-old-daughter) has got sharing, you know, every Monday and Wednesday. It's nothing profound, but, if they didn't share about our family, that would be sad. And, to be closeted, that would be really hard for my kids. Just like if I was closeted, it would be really hard for (my partner) and I.

Similarly, Chandra shows a remarkable ability to manage her life when she describes her current work situation:

> It was eight to five, and now I do nine to two, so that allows me to drive the kids to school, and pick them up, and get dinner going, and make the doctor appointments. All my doctor appointments

are, like, at three or four and I can take them myself. And talk to the teachers and whatever. Plus, I'm off. I teach, so I'm off, too, the same holidays as the kids are.

Finally, this methodology allowed for the examination of relationships between lesbian mother households and institutions in the social environment in considerable detail and with relative ease. For example, one couple interviewed described their relationships with religion as "tenuous/strained." These women, Angie and Cathy, provide an example of the way in which analysis of the narratives led to development of thematic categories useful in understanding the stressors and supports at the intersection of individual/family/community. Angie, 31, is an at-home mother, who attends a liberal church with her adopted 2-year-old-son, Luke. Her partner, Cathy, 30, refuses to participate in family religious activities. Their interviews reveal important information about their struggle to balance individual needs, family cohesion, and contact with their community. Angie commented:

> We all do better when I go (to church)–but I hate that we don't go together . . . I think Luke should have some ideas about spiritual stuff.

Cathy, in a separate interview, referred to her history of being judged and condemned for her lesbianism as well as her gender non-comformity:

> It's fine that (Angie) goes (to church), but I don't need it or want it in my life. I swore that I'd never go to church again . . .

From these and other comments, a series of descriptors and themes were developed that summarize Angie and Cathy's family experiences with the institution of religion. Figure 2 shows a simplified version of their eco map, which includes the couple's comments about the important stressors and strengths in their relationships with church.

These examples of the applications of the eco map methodology demonstrate the promise of the approach for producing data that are rich in detail, meaningful in the context of the respondents' lives, relatively well-organized, and easily understood. Clearly, the most important role of the researcher who uses this methodology is to facilitate the dissemination of the respondents' narratives as they speak for themselves in describing their challenges and successes.

FIGURE 2. Sample eco map

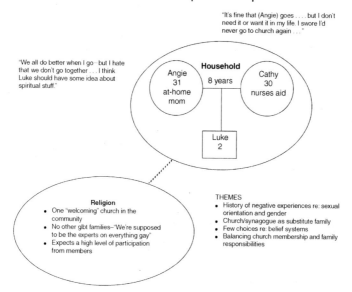

"It's fine that (Angie) goes . . . . but I don't need it or want it in my life. I swore I'd never go to church again . . ."

"We all do better when I go - but I hate that we don't go together . . . I think Luke should have some idea about spiritual stuff."

Household

Angie
31
at-home
mom

8 years

Cathy
30
nurses aid

Luke
2

Religion
- One "welcoming" church in the community
- No other glbt families–"We're supposed to be the experts on everything gay"
- Expects a high level of participation from members

THEMES
- History of negative experiences re: sexual orientation and gender
- Church/synagogue as substitute family
- Few choices re: belief systems
- Balancing church membership and family responsibilities

ENVIRONMENTAL CONTEXT IN THE RESEARCH PROCESS

What better way to study lesbian mothers' relationships within their families and neighborhoods than to interact with these women in their own communities? Next to the use of eco maps to collect and organize data, this project's focus on the environmental context of data collection seemed to contribute most to its success. Understanding how interactions with respondents contributed to knowledge development illustrates these ideas.

The foundation of this study was the relationships that developed between the interviewers and the participants. (And the methodology described here encouraged direct study of respondents in at least one context of their social environments.) Although most lasted only 2-3 hours, these interactions provided the context in which all subsequent data analysis occurred. Most of the interviews took place in respondents' homes, and in most cases, participants offered a tour of the family residence, an invitation for the interviewer to thumb through photo albums, and an introduction to the children. In addition, during the interviews, researchers and participants sat relatively close together, often side-by-side so that the participant could see the eco map and other materials as she spoke. The tone of nearly all interviews paralleled that of a friendly conversation.

Interaction with interview respondents on this level provided interesting detail that might not otherwise be apparent in the data. For example, although many of the interviewees reported incomes that placed them well into the middle class, large variances in indicators of social class other than income were evident. Respondents who reported annual family incomes over $75,000, for example, lived in housing that ranged from a double wide trailer to an historic home in an elegant urban district.

In-home and face-to-face interaction with the interviewees also helped to support the themes evident in the interviews. Observing interactions between mothers and children in their homes and seeing refrigerator doors covered with children's art work and school papers strongly reinforced themes related to mothers' commitment to family and to reports of positive interactions between mothers and children. Seeing the resourcefulness and creativity these women used in remodeling and decorating their homes without outside help gave credence to the idea that they are creative and flexible in other aspects of their lives. Noticing that their neighborhoods were often racially integrated helped make their statements about valuing diversity ring true.

CONCLUSIONS

Eco maps, genograms, and face-to-face interviews are not new tools for social workers. In truth, most of the interview methods described in this paper are likely to be familiar to social work practitioners. Unfortunately, though, the systematic application of these tools to understand women's experiences is relatively uncommon in direct practice and in the study of human behavior and social relationships. In addition, few comprehensive models exist for collecting and organizing these data as they apply to individual, family, and community interactions. This paper proposes one approach to knowledge development that can remedy this weakness in conventional approaches to social research.

By adopting a strategy for data collection with lesbian mothers that accounts for the socio-cultural context in which women live, and by using a data collection tool designed to organize this complex information, we explored the conditions of a group of lesbian mothers in a systematic and inclusive way. Although limited in some ways by the sheer volume of data, this methodology promises to provide information that has important implications for both policy and practice with lesbian mother families. Increased understanding, improved human service practice, and evolved strategies for policy makers are anticipated as benefits of this research model.

Vivid descriptions of social problems naturally flow from studies such as the one described in this paper. Thus, such research has important implications for the development of social policy for minority and oppressed populations. Because the research design derives from an eco-systemic perspective, data flow logically into the arena of social policy since they tend to emphasize social processes, environmental factors, and relationships with institutions. In addition, as highlighted throughout this paper, the feminist research design and philosophy described here emphasizes collaborative relationships between researchers and respondents. These relationships translate easily into social activism and efforts for social justice through political advocacy, program development and public education.

The implications of this research model for direct practice are numerous. Without a doubt, the most valuable aspect of this research model is that it produces data that directly reflect the complex realities of at least a few "real" people who belong to the population being studied. We believe that this condition is vital in bridging the gap between research and practice, in that conclusions drawn from such studies, while not generalizeable, do represent legitimate connection to the lives of women who seek help from practitioners. Another strength of this model is that it avoids unnecessary pathologizing of individuals by placing problems within their social contexts. This strengths-perspective is also evident in the way that this model accentuates the multiple contexts in which individuals and families *successfully* interact with their environments. In our example of lesbian mother families, contextual understanding of these women clearly leads to enhanced sensitivity to potential individual and family needs, and to common developmental and interpersonal experiences.

The methods described in this paper are themselves easily translated into individual work with women. That is, an eco map interview may be used to enhance a comprehensive bio-psycho-social assessment, and the resulting graphic and verbal summary of important relationships may be used to focus problem identification, intervention planning, and the evaluation of treatment efficacy. In short, practitioners who understand the usefulness of exploring the intersections of individuals, families, and communities can use the tools described here to better understand their clients, and to help their clients communicate about–and change–problematic life circumstances.

As the brief examples given here illustrate, research methods that integrate women's voices directly into the study of their lives can be fundamental to the quality and integrity of the research process. When feminist epistemological principles of inclusion and comprehensiveness are carried from data collection to analysis, the results are remarkable for the levels of richness and integration that are reflected in the results. Studies that use this methodology have substantial implications for knowledge development. As with other oppressed populations, few studies of lesbian mothers capture respondents' perspectives on the data collected. Thus, qualitative research of this type is uniquely poised to both support/challenge previous research and suggest areas for important future research. In particular, data analysis can be focused across a sample, as well as within individual narratives in order to yield information about women's lives across individual, family, and community/organizational interactions.

NOTE

1. All names and identifying information have been changed.

REFERENCES

Berardo, F. (1991). Family research in the 1980s: Recent trends and future directions. In A. Booth (Ed.), *Contemporary families: Looking forward, looking back* (pp. 1-11). Minneapolis: National Council on Family Relations.

Bronfenbrenner, U. (1979). *The ecology of human development: Experiments by nature and design.* Boston: Harvard University Press.

Carter, E., & McGoldrick, M. (1980). *The family life cycle: A framework for family therapy.* NY: Gardner Press.

Demo, D., & Allen, K. (1996). Diversity within lesbian and gay families: Challenges and implications for family theory and research. *Journal of Social and Personal Relations, 13 (3),* 44-53.

Feree, M. (1991). Beyond separate spheres: Feminism and family research. In A. Booth (Ed.), *Contemporary families: Looking forward, looking back* (pp. 103-121). Minneapolis: National Council on Family Relations.

Germain, C. (1981). The ecological approach to people-environment transactions. *Social Casework, 62 (6),* 323-331.

Harding, S. (1991). *Whose science? Whose knowledge?* Ithaca: Cornell University Press.

Harold, R., Mercier, L., & Colarossi, L. (1997). Eco maps: A tool to bridge the practice-research gap. *Journal of Sociology and Social Welfare, 24 (4)*, 29-44.

Harold, R., Palmiter, M., Lynch, S., Freedman-Doan, C., & Eccles, J. (2000). Telling the family story: The process. In R. Harold, (Ed.), *Becoming a family: Parent's stories and their implications for practice, research and policy.* Mahwah, NJ: Lawrence Erlbaum and Associates.

Hartman, A. (1978). Diagrammatic assessment of family relationships. *Social Casework, 59*, 465-476.

Jayaratne, T., & Stewart, A. (1991). Quantitative and qualitative methods in the social sciences: Current feminist issues and practical strategies. In M. Fodow & J. Cook, (Eds.), *Beyond methodology: Feminist scholarship as lived research* (pp. 85-106). Indianapolis: Indiana University Press.

McGoldrick, M., & Gerson, R. (1985). Genograms in family assessment. NY: Norton.

Reinharz, S. (1992). *Feminist methods in social research.* New York: Oxford University Press.

Smith, D. (1990). *The conceptual practices of power: A feminist sociology of knowledge.* Boston: Northeastern University Press.

Stacey, J., & Thorne, B. (1985). The missing feminist revolution in sociology. *Social Problems, 32*, 301-316.

Strauss, A., & Corbin, J. (1990). *Basics of qualitative research.* Newbury Park, CA: Sage.

Exit from Poverty:
How "Welfare Mothers"
Achieve Economic Viability

Pamela A. Strother

SUMMARY. There is a large body of research about the characteristics of people in poverty with regard to demographic structures, social stratification, and income differentials, but the processes by which poor people accomplish improvement in their economic situations is a neglected area of the research. Using qualitative procedures, data analysis of interviews with nineteen AFDC-dependent female heads-of-households who received public assistance for at least five consecutive years between 1970 and 1990, and who exited both public assistance and poverty by means other than marriage or cohabitation, resulted in the emergence of a three-part success configuration. Paradoxically, the subjects' concerns were not primarily about exiting welfare, but rather were focused on

Pamela A. Strother, PhD, LCSW, engages in clinical social work practice and administration, provides consultation to government agencies, and conducts trainings for educational, cultural, environmental, and human service organizations.

Address correspondence to: Pamela A. Strother, 411 Catherine Street, Key West, FL 33040.

The study was supported in part by the 1990-91 Blackey Memorial Fellowship from the National Center for Social Policy and Practice.

This article is derived from the author's dissertation research at the School of Social Welfare, State University of New York at Albany.

[Haworth co-indexing entry note]: "Exit from Poverty: How 'Welfare Mothers' Achieve Economic Viability." Strother, Pamela A. Co-published simultaneously in *Journal of Human Behavior in the Social Environment* (The Haworth Social Work Practice Press, an imprint of The Haworth Press, Inc.) Vol. 7, No. 3/4, 2003, pp. 97-119; and: *Women and Girls in the Social Environment: Behavioral Perspectives* (ed: Nancy J. Smyth) The Haworth Social Work Practice Press, an imprint of The Haworth Press, Inc., 2003, pp. 97-119. Single or multiple copies of this article are available for a fee from The Haworth Document Delivery Service [1-800-HAWORTH, 9:00 a.m. - 5:00 p.m. (EST). E-mail address: docdelivery@haworthpress.com].

http://www.haworthpress.com/store/product.asp?sku=J137
Digital Object Identifier: 10.1300/J137v7n03_07

broader life goals more in keeping with the aspirations of those in the economic mainstream. Applications of the findings to social work direct practice focus on the challenges of understanding clients' perceptions and supporting their goals, while dispelling the persistent myths about the poor. Applications to social welfare policy focus on the need to differentiate between public assistance receipt and poverty and to develop policy initiatives that would allow increased monetary assistance to the poor. *[Article copies available for a fee from The Haworth Document Delivery Service: 1-800-HAWORTH. E-mail address: <docdelivery@haworthpress. com> Website: <http://www.HaworthPress.com> © 2003 by The Haworth Press, Inc. All rights reserved.]*

KEYWORDS. Welfare, poverty, single mothers

INTRODUCTION

Single Mothers on Welfare and Single Mothers in Poverty: Two Different Issues

When we talk about welfare mothers leaving the public assistance rolls under the new "welfare reform" mandates, usually no attempt is made to find out what becomes of them once they are no longer on the public dole. The current political climate assumes that getting off welfare is a good thing, when in reality it is often good only for government coffers and rarely positive for the women and children involved. The debate about "welfare reform" is often couched in terms of reducing poverty, but moving off the public welfare[1] rolls is not synonymous with leaving poverty. It is quite possible to exit from welfare through a variety of means and still be thousands of dollars per year below the official federal poverty floor. Even with the recent increase in the minimum wage, a fully employed minimum-wage worker earns $6750 per year *less* than the year 2000 federal poverty level of $17,050 for a family of four. Further, while the increases in the Earned Income Tax Credit provisions have somewhat ameliorated this economic shortfall, the maximum credit for families with more than one qualifying child still does not lift the family out of poverty (U.S. House, Committee on Ways and Means [USCWM], 1998).

The objective of the present climate of welfare reform is not to reduce the poverty rate but to reduce government spending. Policy concerns tend to focus on the size of government transfers to female-headed households. Aid to Families with Dependent Children (AFDC)[2] benefit expenditures have increased 21 percent, after adjusting for inflation, during the period 1970-1996, up to $20.4 billion. During the same period, the real value of AFDC declined by more than 50 percent, with the average monthly benefit for a family of four in 1996 being $374 (USCWM, 1998). While AFDC spending is a small fraction of the federal budget, it became, beginning in the Reagan years, an increasing percentage of state and local budgets (USCWM, 1998). Bringing these increases closer to home has perhaps magnified their impact and has aroused the concern and enmity of many local communities. Public assistance programs are designed to aid those with the lowest incomes from experiencing further destitution (Northrop, 1991), and in no state does the combination of AFDC and food stamps bring family income up to the official poverty line (Will, 1993). Therefore, it is important to make the distinction between the objective of reducing poverty and the objective of reducing government spending. The literature is sorely lacking in attention to the *process* by which people succeed in exiting public assistance *and* attaining non-poverty economic status.

Poverty and Single Mothers

The overall increase, since the early 1980s, of the incidence of poverty of single mothers rearing minor dependent children is reflected in several interrelated factors: increases in numbers of female-headed households; increases in the poverty rates of female headed households; the increasing percentage of children reared in these households[3] (Sawhill, 1988; USCWM, 1998); and the overrepresentation of African Americans, a generally less advantaged demographic group, as female heads of households (Kimenyi, 1991; Sawhill, 1988).

The Spells of Poverty in Female-Headed Households

Two large-scale studies (Bane & Ellwood, 1986; Kniesner, McElroy, & Wilcox, 1988), using two extensive but different databases, have explored the conditions necessary for entry into and exit out of poverty, the so-called "spells" of poverty. For both African Americans and Caucasians, nearly all first observed poverty spells commenced with a change in family structure, not reductions in income within a family structure. Marriage clearly helps keep women out of poverty. The dominant exit mode was (re)marriage or joining the household of another.

The Kniesner data show that the bulk of female-headed family poverty is new poverty, neither carried over from a woman's prior family status nor transmitted to her subsequent family status. Further, leaving female head-of-household poverty means escaping poverty entirely for 60 percent of the African American women and 75 percent of the Caucasian women, not merely experiencing poverty under a different family structure.

The Spells of Welfare in Female-Headed Households

To explore welfare entries and exits, as distinct from poverty entries and exits, Bane and Ellwood (1994) sampled female heads-of-households with children to explore the spells of welfare receipt experienced by the subjects and the beginning and ending events for AFDC receipt. These events mirror, to a large extent, the dynamics of poverty entries and exits. As with the general poverty population, the majority of first entries into the welfare system began when a wife became female head or an unmarried woman without a child became a family head with a child. Exits by means other than (re)marriage or joining another household were due largely to increased earnings of the female head-of-household. The factors that appear to most influence earnings exits are, not surprisingly, education and previous work experience. This is particularly true for those who exit with moderate earnings which may, in some cases, also allow them to exit poverty. Almost 10 percent were unidentified exits, most likely comprised of a combination of administratively-induced ineligibility and recipient choice to discontinue receipt, due to onerous requirements,[4] even though eligible. Return rates fall sharply after two years with no welfare receipt, and, after three years, recidivism is unlikely. The influence of race on welfare spells, when all other factors are held constant, was found to be quite modest.

THE PROCESS OF EXITING

What is it that enables AFDC-dependent female heads-of-households to improve their economic situations so that they are no longer poor?[5] This paper describes a qualitative study that probed the actions and attitudes of women who had not only "gotten off welfare," but who were able to exit poverty as well. Beginning with the methodology of the study and moving through the analysis of the women's experiences and decisions which resulted in the determinants of their successes, the paper culminates in some suggestions for social work interventions in the realms of both human behavior and the social environment.

Who Are These Women?

Located and interviewed from 1990 to 1992, 19 women who received public assistance for five years, the median number of years for durations of poverty spells (Bane & Ellwood, 1994; Sawhill, 1988), were found through contacting agencies, institutions, the media, and personal contacts. At the time of the interviews, the eldest was 59 years old, the youngest was 32, and all were residents of New York State. Fifteen were Caucasian and four were African-American. The number of children per woman ranged from one to six. Fifteen of the women still had at least one child at home for whom they were financially responsible. Most of the women had suffered neglect and/or abuse, physical, sexual, verbal or emotional, some from childhood onward, at the hands of parents, step-parents, foster parents, siblings, spouses, or significant others. Many had been either addicts themselves or members of families in which addiction or mental illness was present.

The comparability of the subjects to the general welfare population is very consistent. Using the data from a large scale study of welfare recipients in Wisconsin (Rank, 1994), the similarities in the attitudes and experiences of the women in both studies indicate that the women in this study are typical of the wider welfare population, suggesting that their behaviors and attitudes are predictive of what enables "average" welfare recipients to exit poverty.

Data collection was done through tape recording face-to-face interviews. Questions were asked of the subjects in the categories of present life circumstances, family of origin and childhood, marriage/couple/children history, health history, education history, employment history, correctional system history, social supports, public assistance history and experience, the history and experience of exiting poverty, self-evaluation and ideas about life in the future, so as to capture as many possibilities for exploration as possible. Observing the time-honored social work maxim of "beginning where the client is," the interviews began with general questions and comments and became more focused as the interview progressed, thus putting questions about potentially stressful subjects later in the interview process.

The audio tapes were then transcribed on computer disks by an out-of-state transcription service to safeguard any possible breach of confidentiality. The interviews resulted in compiling a data bank diverse enough to select from it pertinent incidents[6] relevant to the research question. These incidents then became the material under scrutiny from which the categories for analysis were formed. Following the grounded theory approach (Glaser, 1978; Glaser & Strauss, 1967; Strauss, 1987; Strauss & Corbin, 1990), all the data were first coded, then ordered into preliminary categories according to their conceptual context, and next constantly compared within a category to establish consistency, and across categories to establish both boundaries and interrelatedness. Issues of intensity, frequency, and contingency were explored.

Simultaneous with the process of initial coding was the process of making interpretations and formulations about the various categories in an attempt to discern linkages and interrelationships between and among incidents within a category and between and among the preliminary categories themselves. Analysis of the content of these preliminary categories led to the development of core categories at a higher level of abstraction, which became the major themes and concluding propositions about all the data.

Throughout analysis, HyperResearch, a HyperCard-based, Macintosh application (ResearchWare, Inc., 1993), was used for the storage, coding, organization, retrieval, and analysis of coded materials. Since this author, as the sole researcher, was the only one developing codes and identifying themes, two faculty-recommended students at the State University of New York, College at Oneonta, were retained as coders to establish reliability of coding. A reliability rate of 87% was obtained.

The Experiences of the Women with Employment and Education

Work and schooling are generally believed to be powerful predictors of economic status. Employment experience is often considered a protection against the need for public assistance. All of the women worked at some sort of employment prior to marriage and/or having children. Their jobs ranged from professional positions to blue collar jobs to the military to selling illicit drugs. Almost all of the women, from childhood onward, aspired to a better life via education and employment. Eight of the women (42%) had jobs as children or adolescents. All reported being expected to "work around the house" doing chores and/or supervising younger siblings. Whether they worked inside or outside of the home, all of the women considered themselves to have behaved in a "responsible" manner with regard to their tasks.

All 19 of the women had at least a high school diploma or the equivalent. Three (15.7%) had completed some college work, seven (36.8%)

held two year degrees, two (10.5%) held four year degrees, two had some credits toward master's degrees, and two held master's degrees and doctorates. It should be noted, however, that education alone was not a protection against becoming and/or remaining a welfare recipient. Six (31.5%) had at least some college education and three of those six had degrees when they became recipients. Moreover, one woman, despite having a bachelor's degree and having exited both welfare and poverty once, had returned to the public assistance rolls due to being unable to find a job. By contrast, three of the women had not gone beyond high school but had still achieved enough economic improvement to exit poverty. Several felt that education beyond two years of college was absolutely essential to obtaining living wage employment. This would seem to be borne out by the salaries of the women in this study who held two year degrees–salaries in the $12,000-$15,000 range for years 1988-90, as compared to the women who held bachelor's degrees or higher, who had salaries in the $25,000-$42,000 range.

Experiences with the Welfare System and Exiting Poverty

Despite popular concepts about "intergenerational welfare," less than one-third of the women had received public assistance as part of another household prior to becoming a female head. The remainder reported they had never envisioned themselves being on public assistance.

Yet all the women felt forced, however reluctantly, to seek public assistance when they were unable to support themselves and their children, because either they could not work or their own employment income was insufficient. Twelve of the women (63%) sought public assistance because receiving support from the fathers of their children often proved difficult or impossible:

> It was always difficult to go to Social Services . . . it was always difficult to go to Family Court. Every time I had to do one of those things, as soon as I got to the county office building I had to go to the bathroom . . . my stomach would just churn with all that stuff. But I had two kids and I had a husband who was not dealing with his responsibility . . . so I had to do something. (Muriel)

The thought that they were little different from the welfare department workers except in economic circumstance was one of the major coping mechanisms the women used to ease what they described as the "humiliating" difficulties of receiving public assistance:

> I'd go down to welfare and I'd sit there in the office and I'd see these sloppy women and these lazy, fat men and you know, just what people typically think of as welfare people . . . I shuddered . . . I was in a different category . . . I looked more like the caseworkers. I always looked nice. (Sara)

All the women reported being willing to take whatever steps necessary to secure the public assistance benefits for which they were eligible for themselves and their children, whether they were treated well or badly by the workers. More than half of the women discussed preparing for recertification by keeping all their documentation in special places and dressing appropriately for the occasion:

> I always had exactly what they needed. I had my welfare folder in my alligator bag (laughter) . . . Everything I had always stayed in that bag. I never had to look for anything, nothing was ever missing . . . I used to get dressed up. I went up there like I was going for a business meeting. I would always dress my best . . . like business clothes. (Rita)

Practicing this combination of assertiveness, perseverance, and organization in the face of adversity proved to be a transferable skill for the women, which they used in other difficult situations in their lives.

For 13 women (68.4%) exiting public assistance and exiting poverty occurred simultaneously, because they were able to secure jobs, which provided wages above the poverty level. Some received transitional benefits such as Medicaid, food stamps, and subsidized child care for periods up to nine months following the cessation of their cash grants. Those six women who exited public assistance but whose employment did not immediately lift them out of poverty worked at a vast array of jobs for periods of time ranging from one to ten years between the time they no longer received a public assistance cash grant and the time they earned an income that exceeded the poverty level. All but one of the women received Medicaid and food stamps during this interim period.

At the time of the interviews, most of the women were employed in the human services or in educational settings, many in administrative capacities. One was working in the private-sector. Two were unemployed by choice. One had returned to receiving full public assistance, but continued to be persistent in her search for a living-wage job.

The Women and Their Children

Considering that poverty is often cited as causative to children becoming involved in serious legal and/or emotional difficulties, it would appear that, despite their levels of economic deprivation, the absence and/or instability of romantic relationships, and the lack of parental input from most of the fathers of their children, the women nurtured and protected their children quite well. None of their children had been in serious trouble. Many attended college. Of those who have reached adulthood, all but one were working. Some have married and become parents. None are public assistance recipients.

THE SUCCESS CONFIGURATION

Driving Force, Social Supports, and Opportunity

The women in the study were a diverse group in terms of family of origin, race and ethnicity, levels of health, education and employment, and attachment and behaviors in romantic relationships, and in child rearing. Data analysis revealed a configuration of determinants, common to all the women, that are relevant to their processes of exiting public assistance and poverty. These determinants, the presence of a driving force in their lives, the ability to develop supportive relationships and to participate in community, and the ability to take advantage of opportunity, comprise the success configuration which has enabled them to attain their non-poverty status.

Driving Force: The Heart of the Pursuit

Driving force is the aspect of the woman's life around which all else is organized. It is an overarching objective that subsumes all other conflicts and pursuits. It is both more intense and less specific than pursuing a goal and not necessarily time-limited. It emerges spontaneously, can't be prescribed, and may have been with the woman before or after receipt of public assistance.

Driving force creates a sense of purpose in life to chart a course of action, and maintain it, over a period of time. All of the women in the study had such an area of driving force in which they persevered despite obstacles, using the ability to plan and set incremental goals leading to their objective and doing what is necessary to achieve those goals.

The women discussed driving force as being motivated to accomplish an all-consuming desired objective. Six of the women (31.5%) said that a deliberate decision to remain on AFDC was actually a part of their overall plans to achieve a specific educational or career goal. Of her educational experience, Joan said:

> It was great! I was hooked . . . It wasn't so much the subject matter, but here was this batch of legally employed lunatics, the professors, who were very similar to me. A support group materialized. I worked incredibly hard . . . I was running on sheer determination a lot of the time. I was staying up late typing papers . . . I can't miss these classes. I got paranoid about it . . . I would wake up not knowing when I was going to get to college because my car wouldn't start and some days it just quit and I would just end up walking [a distance of almost ten miles one way] . . . But I was determined. That's just how I do it. I think that just wanting to get off welfare isn't enough. You have to want to work your ass off.

In terms of pursuing her career as a human services professional, Cicely said:

> I wasn't thinking about the salary being enough to get me out of poverty. It was about my own salary, my own job, my own office. I had never had this. Being with professionals, helping people. That was my thought. [Exiting AFDC] wasn't the most important thing.

Others chose to remain on public assistance in order to be with their children, particularly in the absence of fathers' involvement with the children.

> [Staying on public assistance] was a deliberate decision because I felt that it was more important for me to put in the time with the children when they were small than to pursue a career. Because it was really hard when I was trying to work and dragging my little kids back and forth to a babysitter and then when you come home you were tired and you just wanted to put them to bed and not think about them . . . You know, I had to stay home with these children. (Kim)

Two (10.5%) continued public assistance to pursue spiritual goals, e.g., recovery from active alcoholism and devotion to a religious ministry.

Surprisingly, "getting off welfare" was not the driving force for any of the women. Whatever difficulties the women encountered as public assistance recipients, these women underscored the futility of taking a minimum wage job with no benefits only to find oneself worse off economically than when receiving public assistance. In response to the question about what advice she'd give a woman on public assistance, Alice said, "I would tell her to use her time to develop the skills that are necessary to get a job that is more than minimum wage ... get some education in a field that's going to help you find a good paying job afterward." Bonnie added the advice that the woman should not be intimidated and thus deterred from her goal. " ... [I]t was a lot of harassment. You know, 'you have to get off it [public assistance] ... because we're [the caseworkers] not going to wait around for you' [to finish school]."

All of the women used the word "goal" frequently in their conversations. They spoke about the ways in which they planned, developed goals, and overcame obstacles to achieving those goals. This ability was present before they were public assistance recipients and may be accounted for in part by their capacity to engage in abstract thinking and organizational skills. Incrementalism was mentioned by many of the women as the way that they accomplished their planning and goal-setting without becoming overwhelmed. Muriel was typical of the women when she said, "I need to break things down into small pieces that feel manageable to me ... I don't have to make a decision about finishing the whole thing."

All of the women spoke of planning in terms of budgeting monies and prioritizing payments and purchases, using elaborate systems of envelopes, cigar boxes, and checking and savings accounts, in their on-going attempts to maintain financial stability while pursuing their goals. However, not all planning and goal-setting revolved around money. Some women "used the system" to better themselves economically by "researching" rules and regulations so that they could use them legally to their advantage. One of the women, in conjunction with other people in her church community, started an after school program two years before her child went to school, so that she would have a place with which she was comfortable to leave her daughter when she went back to work. Other non-monetary planning and goal-setting included hunting wild game for food, vegetable gardening and raising chickens, and home sewing to provide clothing. "I'm always planning ... you do what you have to do to reach your goal . . . I don't want anything screwing up my goals," Liz said.

Although not always successful, attempting to have savings in some form, usually cash, but also food stamps, and store layaway programs, was seen by all the women as an important component of reaching one's goals. Because public assistance regulations do not permit the accumulation of cash savings, they hid their assets under the names of relatives or in dresser drawers. The cash savings were accomplished in small increments:

> . . . I would save a little bit here and there from each check and I'd take it down to the parent's house and put it in the freezer in this little cup . . . Whatever it was. If it was $10 or $20 or maybe $50 during the summer months. . . [when] there wasn't as much need for fuel . . . You didn't eat as much in the summertime . . . And I saved $800 [over a 15 month period] . . . because in the back of my mind I knew . . . the car isn't going to last forever . . . You live out here in the boonies. You don't have a car. Then I would really be dependent on my parents. (Noreen)

Upon exit from public assistance, having some "emergency" money was cited by the women as a factor in not being a welfare recidivist as they struggled to gain financial equilibrium.

No matter how intense one's driving force may be, the capacity to persevere toward one's goal despite obstacles is necessary to bring it to fruition. Many of the women cited problems with fatigue, depression, physical and mental illness, acute stress, boredom, and discouragement at times during their quests to realize their driving force goals, and hope was mentioned repeatedly by the women as part of their capacity to persevere. They also spoke of the planning they had done that had not worked out as they had intended, e.g., failures with cross-country relocations, abortive attempts at education, disappointments in seeking employment opportunities, and futile attempts to save money and plan financially for pregnancies and births in an effort to avoid becoming welfare recipients. The African American women in the study felt it was particularly important to persevere in the face of racial bias. Sandy echoed the thoughts of the others by offering this advice to women still receiving public assistance:

Don't give up. Keep your eye on what's important to you, what you really want to do. Keep thinking about it until you can figure out how to go about it. Don't let setbacks destroy you. Never give up.

The Women and Support Systems: "I Get By with a Little Help from My Friends"

Throughout the interviews, the women used phrases about "support systems," in the sense of having a variety of people on whom they could rely. The ability to develop supportive relationships allowed the women to garner emotional sustenance and to increase their own tangible and intangible resources, factors all of them cited as being instrumental in their exit from public assistance and poverty. Even when her family and friends were as poor as the woman herself, help in the form of sharing shelter, food, and companionship made a difference.

Participation in community included being active in religious, volunteer, and social groups, and in taking advantage of networking opportunities, e.g., hearing about jobs, child care, housing, entitlements, cultural and recreational activities, and social programs. Many also felt that the support of mentors and counselors enabled them to remain in educational or vocational programs dealing successfully with multiple difficulties while attending school:

> She was not only my therapist, she was my mentor. She had done a lot of things that weren't traditional for women. Or she was doing them . . . [she was] the catalyst for finding out and getting out of that situation [of being physically abused]. (Cheryl)

Spirituality was mentioned by the women as a social and emotional support. This sense of "invisible support," as well as the feeling that "help" was available from some "greater source," should not be overlooked as a factor which sustained the women. The presence of spirituality and faith in some universal scheme of things was mentioned by all of the women as something that had helped them endure the vicissitudes of their lives and proceed toward their short- and long-term goals. While not always conceived as a recognized religion, each woman pursued a spiritual path to which she was committed and in which she found solace and strength.

Opportunity: "Take It Where You Find It"

The women had a strong capacity for recognizing those opportunities that would further their driving force goals. They got information through fliers, bulletin boards, coworkers, and acquaintances. They were willing to pursue opportunity when it arose, and again, as with planning and goal-setting, stressed the desirability of taking advantage of opportunity in an incremental manner, as well as the ability to tolerate uncertainty, such as accepting temporary employment, not knowing if it would lead to permanent employment. Each of the women had some access to the economic mainstream through contacts with resources such as family, friends, and educational or human service programs. Because they were not "ghettoized" in terms of being exposed only to others who were as disadvantaged as they, a greater range of opportunities presented themselves, not just for increased income but for other opportunities as well.

Perhaps because of their participation in supportive social relationships, these women were able to be verbally assertive, to "speak up," to those figures in authority who might be able to assist them in providing opportunities. Most of the women remembered with gratitude opportunities presented to them by others that were beyond what was expected. These opportunities were often the result of someone in a position of authority "bending the rules," while expecting nothing in return, so that the woman could achieve a desired goal.

Not all of the opportunities that presented themselves were legitimate. Eight of the women (42%) said that they had engaged in activities that were forbidden by public assistance regulations. These infractions involved gaining additional income while continuing to receive cash grants, but only four of the women (21%) worked covertly while receiving assistance:

> I'm not taking from nobody with a side job under the table. Although the system, if they knew I was, they would have cut me off, you know. I had nobody. I had no relatives and I knew that I had to do something for my child and myself. She should not be denied of things because she only has me. And that's how I justified doing a little extra work. (Terry)

Many of the women believed that the public assistance system is one which encourages fraud with its stinginess and punitive regulations:

> ... [O]ne of the things on welfare is that you learn that you have lots of choices with them but most of them mean you have to be able to manipulate. ... It's not that it makes you feel proud to do this to the system, it's that the system can give you no alternatives. (Marilyn)

In summary, many of the areas often considered pertinent when examining reasons for human behavior, such as family-of-origin, family-of-choice, race and ethnicity, education, and health, yielded little that was consistent among the women. However, the three-part success configuration which enabled the women to obtain economically viable and emotionally satisfying life situations is in many aspects similar to mechanisms employed by the non-poor segment of society. Overall, the interests of these women were broader than just economic concerns. They felt that they could not successfully pursue goals that were not their own, such as getting any job or leaving their children, merely to exit public assistance. The implications of this perspective can be instructive to the social work profession when dealing with "welfare mothers," as well as other categories of low-income clients.

CHALLENGES TO PROFESSIONAL SOCIAL WORK WITH THE POOR

Understanding the Client's Reality and Dispelling the Myths

Many of the rules, regulations, practices and pressures put on welfare recipients by the public assistance system are obstacles to attaining economic viability which would be thought ridiculous if applied to mainstream society (Ellwood, 1988; Handler & Hasenfeld, 1991; Sherraden, 1991). Considered within a person-in-environment perspective, public assistance recipients are often subjected to disincentives so extreme that simple survival at both the economic and emotional levels saps their strength and there is none left for exiting pursuits. Social workers must understand that these disincentives are based on ideological arguments about poverty and welfare. Such arguments ignore a growing body of research which refutes the myths about the poor in general and public assistance recipients in particular.

The Culture of Poverty Myth: Social welfare policy, historically and contemporarily, assumes that low income people don't have the appropriate dominant culture values in such areas as work and family life (Handler, 1995; Handler & Hasenfeld, 1991). The poor are thus perceived as deviant and must therefore be compelled and coerced to conform to the mores of the middle class. However, Galbraith (1979, 1983) points out that attitudes of the poor vary little from those of other social classes. Rank (1994) found that the welfare recipients in his sample held "fundamental American values." The women in this study generally held the same kinds of values, as reflected in their behaviors and beliefs, as those held by the dominant culture, as well as a variety of characteristics which were relevant to their successful outcomes, e.g., adequate intellective capacity for abstract thinking and reasoning, an awareness of one's environment, the ability to plan and set goals and persevere toward those goals despite obstacles and problems, and the ability to exercise adult-appropriate levels of autonomy. They made positive choices in terms of neighborhoods and housing, schools for their children, pursuit of their own education and employment, and financial planning and obligations.

Unlike those in better economic circumstances, choice for recipients under the present system is often severely limited. Present public assistance regulations prohibit recipients from doing what many people who lead economically viable lives do: getting help from others in the forms of loans of money, barters, favors, and other supports from family and friends. In addition, "incentives" in programs for the poor often don't work because such incentives are not based on individual choice and are not congruent with the person's sense of her own direction, e.g., offering education as an incentive to exit public assistance to a woman whose driving force is remaining at home with preschool children.[7] Despite these tremendous obstacles, the women in this study followed their own internal sense of their appropriate life paths and negotiated the public assistance system in ways that moved them along their chosen route, often modeling the mores of the dominant middle class culture.

In addition, the women cited the necessity of considering those areas of human motivation which are difficult to define and to quantify when looking for solutions to human problems: the importance of informal and formal social networks and programs of social support, including the intangible, but critical, support of spiritual sustenance, as well as the maintenance of hope. In working with clients, social workers must recognize that continued experiences of isolation and futility, which segregate low income mothers from middle class types of opportunity, often have a negative impact on both the hope and the motivation of the poor.

The Dependency Myth: The focus of the welfare "problem" has shifted in the past twenty-five years from alleviating poverty to alleviating dependency (Abramovitz, 1996; Danziger, 1989; Murray, 1984; Novak, 1988; Piven & Cloward, 1987), in response to a policy climate that has become increasingly hostile to the persistently poor population. Political rhetoric often clouds the "welfare issue" so that reducing the numbers of people receiving welfare and reducing the incidence of poverty are presented as being synonymous, when they are not. The major intent of present welfare policy is to reduce the costs of the public assistance system in federal, state and local budgets, not to reduce poverty. Even the federal government has concluded that, despite savings in public dollars due to decreased eligibility and benefits in welfare programs, poverty, regardless of the measure of income used, has increased substantially over the past 15 years (USCWM, 1998). A recent study about the well-being of former welfare recipients (Cancian et al., 1999) found that, for women who had to depend solely on their own incomes, 64 percent were still poor five years after AFDC exit. The study concluded that this was due in part to the current reforms which force women with fewer employment prospects to leave the rolls when the opportunities for living wage employment may not be available to them.

Income disparity has also increased dramatically, beginning in 1980 (Abramovitz, 1996; Krugman, 1990; Michel, 1991; Sawhill, 1989). As of 1996, the latest year for which figures are available, an all-time high of 49.2 percent of income was concentrated in the top quintile of the population, while the income of the bottom quintile had declined to an all time low of 3.6 percent (U.S. Bureau of the Census, 1998; USCWM, 1998). This downward shift in income for a large proportion of the population perhaps has led to directing increased hostility toward those on welfare, as former members of the middle class who are now in a lower-income class react to their contracted economic situations. It is easier to label a public assistance recipient "dependent" than to look at the major structural change required to create conditions and opportunities for employment which will produce incomes securely and comfortably distant from the poverty line (Northrup, 1991).

The Disinclination to Work Myth: Decades of inquiry refute stereotypes concerning patterns of dependency and disinclination to work (Chambre, 1985; Chrissinger, 1980; Duncan, 1984; Goodwin, 1972; Harris, 1993; Levitan & Johnson, 1984; Macarov, 1970; Rein & Rainwater, 1977). The underpinning of our present public assistance policy remains the moral imperative established by the Elizabethan Poor Laws: work and work training for the able-bodied, retooling for the unemployed, and workfare and minimal support for those who cannot work. Work policies and programs persist in various forms despite overwhelming historical and contemporary evidence that they fail to reduce the welfare rolls in any appreciable way or to improve the economic self-sufficiency of the poor (Handler & Hasenfeld, 1991). A recent report by the Manpower Demonstration Research Corporation said that, while the effects of the JOBS Programs differed across states, as many as 68 percent of participants in the JOBS Programs remained on AFDC (USCWM, 1998), and a Congressional Research Service report concluded that even those AFDC recipients who found work might still be poor despite supplementation by the earned income credit (USCWM, 1998). An analysis of Wisconsin AFDC data (Cancian et al., 1999) found that only one-third of women who exited welfare achieved the income level they had received just prior to exiting AFDC. The fact that the women in the study felt it was wiser to remain on public assistance in order to have a better lifestyle than if they were working at a minimum-wage or other low paying job is *not* an indictment of the women's industry but of an economy that provides work at which one cannot make a living. The strategy of the new welfare "reform" of reducing benefit levels or removing recipients from the rolls through excessive sanctions, in order to make minimum wage or other low paying jobs more attractive, must be questioned in terms of the degeneration of economic and social viability of the families affected.

CONCLUSION

The present "welfare reform" commits the same errors as other reforms over the past six hundred years (Handler, 1995). If we pay attention to the experiences of the women in this study, one of the potential changes in direction for the domestic welfare programs might be to institute policies that will put more money in poor people's pockets, while creating an atmosphere free of stigma and undue hardship.

A Different Answer: Putting More Cash in the Hands of the Poor

Living Wage Employment: The point was amply made by the study's participants, who chose to remain on public assistance rather than take a minimum wage job, that the minimum wage is still woefully inadequate despite the recent and proposed changes. A single mother with three children would have to work one full-time and one half-time job under the present minimum wage to lift her family just barely out of poverty, all the while simultaneously rearing children and overseeing a household. In order to exceed the year 2000 federal poverty guidelines, full-time employment (40 hours per week for 50 weeks a year) at a rate of $8.53 an hour would be required. An economy without a sufficient amount of *living wage* employment relative to the numbers of people seeking that employment mitigates against individual economic viability and must be addressed, rather than blaming low-income people for their inability to exit welfare.

Anti-Poverty Insurance: Virtually every woman interviewed spoke in a heartfelt manner about the sense of humiliation and degradation she experienced from the stigma of being a "welfare mother." Instituting a provision for anti-poverty insurance, as opposed to public assistance, as a non-deviant entitlement, in the same way we now regard unemployment insurance or social security and disability insurance would help to increase an individual's sense of self-worth leading to increased motivation to succeed economically. An additional benefit of the use of the anti-poverty insurance concept is that it would enable the existing welfare bureaucracy, in modified form, to be utilized so that unemployment would not be created by dismantling it.

Child Support Collection and Payments: The "beginning event" for entry into the public assistance system as a single mother, for every woman in this study, was her inability to support her children on her own. Often, she did not receive support from the child(ren)'s father(s). This problem has been addressed to a limited degree by child support laws, but enforcement of these laws is often lax and still requires unrealistic effort on the part of the custodial parent. The increased attention to collection of child support for those on public assistance focuses primarily on reimbursing the state for welfare payments,[8] not on increasing available income for women and children (Harris, 1987-88). A public assistance policy to put more of this income into the hands of mothers is needed.

Accumulation of Savings: Having savings was cited by many of the women in the study as a way of guarding against the severity of repeated personal economic decline in the face of unanticipated expenses, which may mean the difference between the continued need for public assistance and the ultimate goal of economic self-sufficiency. In addition, the presence of savings enabled the women to feel some degree of adult-appropriate autonomy and independence. Although present public assistance regulations prohibit the accumulation of savings, the presence of savings in some form enabled the women in the study to have extra resources with which to exit welfare and to guard against welfare recidivism in emergencies. The present policy needs to be altered.

The Mandate for Social Work

The directions to which the conclusions of this study point appear to be at considerable odds with the emerging social welfare policy which is increasingly punitive and mean-spirited. In addition, social workers must guard against becoming enculturated in this negative perception of those on welfare. The social work profession has both an historical and present-day imperative to address the issues of poverty and welfare by (1) taking into consideration the worldview of economically disadvantaged women, (2) bringing about reform in terms of correcting what has been proven to be defective or ineffective, and (3) renewing and expanding its efforts to address the incidence of poverty, not the receipt of welfare, as a major issue for social policy.

The terms public assistance and welfare are used interchangeably to refer to the "package" of benefits received by the women in this study, which includes AFDC grants, Medicaid, and food stamps. When only some portion of public assistance or other types of income maintenance are cited, they will be specifically named.

This study was completed prior to the Personal Responsibility and Work Opportunity Reconciliation Act of 1996, and so does not include discussion of the provisions of Temporary Assistance to Needy Families, which are more stringent than those of AFDC.

Increases in the percentage of children living in poverty appears to stem from an increase in the number of families in poverty rather than an increase in the numbers of children in poor families (Bane & Jargowsky, 1988; Axinn & Hirsch, 1993). More than 88 percent of AFDC families had three or fewer children in 1995. The average family size was 2.8 persons (U.S. House, Committee on Ways and Means, 1998).

For example, several women in this study were asked inappropriate questions about their sexual activity and caseworkers suggested to another woman that she send her seven-year-old son to live with relatives, so that she could rent out his room to gain income.

"Female head-of-household" is defined as a single woman who is the mother of one or more dependent minor children who are living with her in her own household. "AFDC-dependent" is defined as receiving cash income from Aid to Families with Dependent Children for all or part of family/household income for at least five consecutive years between 1970 and 1990, the range of years in which poverty, declines in income, and income inequality grew at an accelerated rate (Sawhill, 1989; Krugman, 1990; Michel, 1991) making life more difficult for those at the lower end of the economic spectrum. "No longer poor" is defined as a household headed by a woman whose own income exceeded federal poverty guidelines for at least two consecutive years between 1970 and 1992.

An incident is defined as any unit of data deemed significant to the study. Therefore an incident could be a feeling or an opinion, as well as an event or a situation.

Presumably there are non-welfare working mothers who may wish to stay home with children, but do not have the economic opportunity to do so. Because economic exigencies create lack of choice in some segments of the population, that is not a reason to build such lack of choice into social policy, but rather a reason to seek to create conditions which make choice available to all.

The recipient gets a maximum of $50 per month of any child support payments as a "pass through." The remainder goes to the child support agency (U.S. House, Committee on Ways and Means, 1998).

NOTES

1. The terms public assistance and welfare are used interchangeably to refer to the "package" of benefits received by the women in this study, which includes AFDC grants, Medicaid, and food stamps. When only some portion of public assistance or other types of income maintenance are cited, they will be specifically named.

2. This study was completed prior to the Personal Responsibility and Work Opportunity Act of 1996, and so does not include discussion of the provisions of Temporary Assistance to Needy Families, which are more stringent than those of AFDC.

3. Increases in the percentage of children living in poverty appears to stem from an increase in the number of families in poverty rather than an increase in the numbers of children in poor families (Bane & Jargowsky, 1988; Axinn & Hirsch, 1993). More than 88 percent of AFDC families had three or fewer children in 1995. The average family size was 2.8 persons (U.S. House, Committee on Ways and Means, 1998).

4. For example, several women in this study were asked inappropriate questions about their sexual activity, and caseworkers suggested to another woman that she send her seven-year-old son to live with relatives, so that she could rent out his room to gain income.

5. "Female head-of-household" is defined as a single woman who is the mother of one or more dependent minor children who are living with her in her own household. "AFDC-dependent" is defined as receiving cash income from Aid to Families with Dependent Children for all or part of family/household income for at least five consecutive years between 1970 and 1990, the range of years in which poverty, declines in income, and income inequality grew at an accelerated rate (Sawhill, 1989; Krugman, 1990; Michel, 1991), making life more difficult for those at the lower end of the economic spe rum, "No longer poor" is defined as a household headed by a woman whose own income exceeded federal poverty guidelines for at least two consecutive years between 1970 and 1992.

6. An incident is defined as any unit of data deemed significant to the study. Therefore, an incident could be a feeling or opinion, as well as an event or a situation.

7. Presumably there are non-welfare working mothers who may wish to stay home with children but do not have the economic opportunity to do so. Because economic

exigencies create lack of choice in some segments of the population, that is not a reason to build such lack of choice into social policy, but rather a reason to seek to create conditions which make choice available to all.

8. The recipient gets a maximum of $50 per month of any child support payments as a "pass through." The remainder goes to the child support agency (U.S. House, Committee on Ways and Means, 1998).

REFERENCES

Abramovitz, M. (1996). *Under attack, fighting back: Women and welfare in the United States.* New York: Monthly Review Press.

Axinn, J., & Hirsch, A. (1993). Welfare and reform of women. *Families in Society, 74,* 563-72.

Bane, M., & Ellwood, D. (1986). Slipping into and out of poverty: The dynamics of spells. *Journal of Human Resources, 21,* 1-23.

Bane, M., & Ellwood, D. (1994). *Welfare realities: From rhetoric to reform.* Cambridge, MA: Harvard University Press.

Bane, M., & Jargowsky, P. (1988). The links between government policy and family structure: What matters and what doesn't. In A.J. Cherlin (Ed.), *The changing American family and public policy* (pp. 219-251). Washington DC: Urban Institute Press.

Cancian, M., Haveman, R., Kaplan, T., Meyer, D., & Wolfe, B. (1999). Work, earnings, and well-being after welfare: What do we know? In Danziger, S. (Ed.) *Economic conditions and welfare reform* (pp.161-186). Kalamazoo, MI: W.E. Upjohn Institute for Employment Research.

Chambre, S. (1985, January). Role orientations and intergenerational welfare use. *Social Casework,* 13-20.

Chrissinger, M. (1980). Factors affecting employment of welfare mothers. *Social Work, 25,* 52-56.

Danziger, S. (1989). Fighting poverty and reducing welfare dependency. In P.H. Cottingham & D.T. Ellwood (Eds.), *Welfare Policy for the 1990s* (pp. 41-69). Cambridge, MA: Harvard University Press.

Duncan, G. (1984). *Years of poverty, years of plenty.* Ann Arbor: University of Michigan, Institute for Social Research, Survey Research Center.

Ellwood, D.T. (1988). *Poor support: Poverty in the American family.* New York: Basic Books, Inc.

Galbraith, K. (1979). *The nature of mass poverty.* Cambridge, MA: Harvard University Press.

Galbraith, K. (1983). *The voice of the poor.* Cambridge, MA: Harvard University Press.

Glaser, B. (1978). *Theoretical sensitivity.* Mill Valley, CA: Sociology Press.

Glaser, B., & Strauss, A. (1967). *The discovery of grounded theory: Strategies for qualitative research.* Chicago: Aldine Publishing Company.

Goodwin, L. (1972). *Do the poor want to work? A social-psychological study of work orientations.* Washington, D.C.: Brookings Institution.

Handler, J.F. (1995). *The poverty of welfare reform: The underclass and antipoverty policy.* New Haven, CT: Yale University Press.

Handler, J.F., & Hasenfeld, Y. (1991). *The moral construction of poverty: Welfare reform in America.* Newbury Park, CA: Sage Publications.

Harris, D. (1987-88). Child support for welfare families. *New York University Review of Law and Social Change, 16,* 713-733.

Harris, K. (1993). Work and welfare among single mothers in poverty. *American Journal of Sociology, 99,* 317-52.

HyperResearch [Computer software]. (1993). Randolph, MA: ResearchWare, Inc.

Kimenyi, M. (1991). Rational choice, culture of poverty, and the intergenerational transmission of welfare dependency. *Southern Economic Journal, 51,* 947-960.

Kniesner, T., McElroy, M., & Wilcox, S. (1988). Getting into poverty without a husband, and getting out, with or without. *The American Economic Review, 78,* 86-90.

Krugman, P. (1990). The income distribution disparity. *Challenge: The Magazine of Economic Affairs, 33,* 4-6.

Levitan, S., & Johnson, C. (1984). *Beyond the safety net: Reviving the promise of opportunity in America.* Cambridge, MA: Ballinger Publishing Company.

Macarov, D. (1970). *Incentives to work.* San Francisco, CA: Jossey-Bass, Inc.

Michel, R. (1991). Economic growth and income equality since the 1982 recession. *Journal of Policy Analysis and Management, 10,* 181-20.

Murray, C. (1984). *Losing ground: American social policy, 1950-1980.* New York: Basic Books.

Northrop, E. (1991). Public assistance and antipoverty programs or why haven't means-tested program been more successful at reducing poverty. *Journal of Economic Issues, XXV,* 1017-27.

Novak, M. (1988). The new war on poverty. *Focus, 11,* 6-10.

Piven, F.F., & Cloward, R. (1987). The contemporary relief debate. In F. Block, R.A. Cloward, B. Ehrenreich, & F.F. Piven (Eds.), *The mean season: The attack on the welfare state* (pp. 45-108). New York: Pantheon Books.

Rank, M.R. (1994). *Living on the edge: The realities of welfare in America.* New York: Columbia University Press.

Rein, M., & Rainwater, L. (1977). How large is the welfare class? *Challenge: The Magazine of Economic Affairs, 20,* 23.

Sawhill, I. (1988). Poverty in the U.S.: Why is it so persistent? *Journal of Economic Literature, XXVI,* 1073-1119.

Sawhill, I. (1989). Reaganomics in retrospect: Lessons for a new administration. *Challenge: The Magazine of Economic Affairs, 32,* 57-59.

Sherraden, M. (1991). *Assets and the poor: A new American welfare policy.* Armonk, NY: M.E. Sharpe, Inc.

Strauss, A. (1987). *Qualitative analysis for social scientists.* Cambridge, MA: Cambridge University Press.

Strauss, A., & Corbin, J. (1990). *Basics of qualitative research: Grounded theory, procedures, and techniques.* Newbury Park, CA: Sage Publications.

U.S. Bureau of the Census. (1998). *Money Income in the United States: 1998. Series P60-206.* Washington, DC: U.S. Government Printing Office.

U.S. House of Representatives. Committee on Ways and Means. (1998). *1998 Green Book: Background Material and Data on Programs Within the Jurisdiction of the Committee on Ways and Means.* Washington, DC: U.S. Government Printing Office.

Will, J. (1993). Public perceptions of the deserving poor. *Social Science Research, 22,* 312-22.

Importance of Macro Social Structures and Personality Hardiness to the Stress-Illness Relationship in Low-Income Women

Dorothy M. Williams

Kathleen A. Lawler

SUMMARY. Individuals confronted with poverty are at increased risk for disease and death due, in part, to the influence of macro social structures on differential exposure and heightened responsiveness to stress (Williams, 1990). For this reason, the influence of personality hardiness in moderating the stress-illness relationship in a biracial sample (African-American and European-American) of low-income women was examined. The effect of differential perceptions of the community on illness also was studied. Participants (100) completed rating scales, including Social Readjustment, Dispositional Resilience, Community Stress, and Seriousness of Illness. Hierarchical regression indicated that

Dorothy M. Williams is affiliated with the School of Social and Community Services, The University of Tennessee, Chattanooga, TN.

Kathleen A. Lawler is affiliated with the Department of Psychology, University of Tennessee, Knoxville, TN.

Address correspondence to: Dorothy Williams, School of Social and Community Services, University of Tennessee, 615 McCallie Avenue, Chattanooga, TN 37403 (E-mail: dorothy-williams@utc.edu).

[Haworth co-indexing entry note]: "Importance of Macro Social Structures and Personality Hardiness to the Stress-Illness Relationship in Low-Income Women." Williams, Dorothy M., and Kathleen A. Lawler. Co-published simultaneously in *Journal of Human Behavior in the Social Environment* (The Haworth Social Work Practice Press, an imprint of The Haworth Press, Inc.) Vol. 7, No. 3/4, 2003, pp. 121-140; and: *Women and Girls in the Social Environment: Behavioral Perspectives* (ed: Nancy J. Smyth) The Haworth Social Work Practice Press, an imprint of The Haworth Press, Inc., 2003, pp. 121-140. Single or multiple copies of this article are available for a fee from The Haworth Document Delivery Service [1-800-HAWORTH, 9:00 a.m. - 5:00 p.m. (EST). E-mail address: docdelivery@haworthpress.com].

hardiness moderated the stress-illness relationship ($p < .01$), with high stress, low hardy women having higher levels of illness. In addition, race moderated the effect of stress, with high stress, Caucasian women having higher levels of illness. Group mean differences on community stress scores for low and high hardy women were obtained ($p < .0001$), but community stress was not associated with illness. Stress is linked to illness in low-income women; furthermore, both personality hardiness and being African-American buffer the effect of stress. *[Article copies available for a fee from The Haworth Document Delivery Service: 1-800-HAWORTH. E-mail address: <docdelivery@haworthpress.com> Website: <http://www.Haworth Press.com>* © *2003 by The Haworth Press, Inc. All rights reserved.]*

KEYWORDS. Stress, women, social class, hardiness, race, health

Women and low-income people are sicker (Thomas, 1997) than are men and higher socioeconomic status individuals. The poor have a lower life expectancy, a higher rate of mortality, and a higher rate of chronic diseases than do middle and upper income individuals (Kessler & McRae, 1981; Marmot, 1994; Marmot, Shipley, & Rose, 1984; Pappas, Queen, Hadden, & Fisher, 1993; Wilkinson, 1992). Women, according to Kaplan, Anderson, and Wingard (as cited in Thomas, 1997) restrict their activities for health problems more than men, lose more well years of life from morbidity, and have higher rates of hospitalization than men. The association between lower socioeconomic status and poorer health was noted in the literature as early as four decades ago. More recent epidemiological studies clearly establish this link and document that socioeconomic differentials in health have both persisted and increased in magnitude (Marmot, 1994; Pappas, Queen, Haden, & Fisher, 1993; Siegrist, 1995). Irrespective of race and sex, greater declines in the direct age-adjusted death rates for higher socioeconomic status individuals than for lower socioeconomic status individuals have been noted in the United States (Pappas et al., 1993). Epidemiological research has established clearly that poverty is a risk factor for physical illness and for psychological distress. Other research has shown that women and African Americans are disproportionately represented among America's poor, thereby placing them at higher risk for health problems (Northrop, 1990). Almost two-thirds of the poor over 16 years of age are female. For African-Americans, the picture is even more dismal. Thirty-five percent of African-Americans live in poverty compared to

13 percent of the general population. Thirty-two percent of African-Americans experience health-related financial difficulties compared with 17 percent of European-Americans, and two to three times more African-Americans than European-Americans experience difficulties affording basic necessities (Blendon et al., 1995). What is it about low socioeconomic status that places individuals at higher risk for disease and death?

The social structure and personality perspective, suggests that since individuals' behaviors and values are shaped by macro environmental structures, SES differentials in health are due, in part, to conditions in life that derive from an individual's "structural position" (Williams, 1990). Based on this view, macro social structures account for both the differential exposure and differential vulnerability of the poor to stressful life events. Life in America's impoverished neighborhoods exposes people to conditions where stressors of material scarcities are compounded by limitations on exercising choice, exposure to high levels of contagion stress, lack of upward mobility, and higher incidences of personal victimization (Belle, 1982; Ingram, Coring, & Schmidt, 1996). In addition, economic deprivation exposes the poor to life in risky neighborhoods where they are continually confronted with dangers, including rats, faulty electrical wring, exposed elevator shafts, broken glass and trash in the streets, gun fire, fighting, and crime. One study (Rainwater, 1970) of life in a federal housing project found that over 50% of the residents expressed concern over exposure to fighting, crime, and substance abuse. Conditions in one's neighborhood have been shown to have a weak but positive correlation with feeling bad and a negative association with feelings of well-being (Cohen, Struening, Genevie, Kaplan, Muhlin, & Peck, 1992). The differential exposure hypothesis proposes that poor people encounter stress producing life events more frequently than their higher socioeconomic status counterparts, and this frequency of exposure to stressors is associated with the higher rates of psychological and physical pathology found among disadvantaged populations. Support for the differential exposure hypothesis comes from the Dohrenwend study (1973), which showed that life change scores for all events, including events probably beyond the respondents' control, were significantly related to SES for the lower socioeconomic status group, but not for the higher socioeconomic status group.

Macro social structures also may account for the differential stress responsiveness of lower socioeconomic status individuals (Williams, 1990). The differential stress vulnerability hypothesis was supported by the Kessler and Cleary study (1980), which found that people of lower socioeconomic status were more likely to experience emotional distress when under stress than were middle and upper status people. Women also have been found to be more vulnerable to stress. However, this greater vulnerability is limited to specific stressors which affect women's relationships, such as the death of a spouse, or to vicarious stress, which is related to people in the social networks of women (Kessler & McLeod, 1984). Thus, social networks that provide support and protection for low-income women are also sources of stress.

The social structure and personality perspective allows for the role of psychosocial factors in the relationship between SES and health. Two major psychosocial factors, stress and coping, are viewed as central determinants of health (Williams, 1990). The stress-illness relationship is well documented in the literature. Causal research models provide ample evidence that physiological changes, relevant to a number of different illnesses, can be induced by physical stressors of varying characteristics, including uncontrollability, unpredictability, chronicity, and severity (Anisman, Pizzino, & Sklar, 1980; Baizman, Cox, Osman, & Goldstein, 1979; Kvetnansky, Kopin, & Saavedra, 1978). Most of these characteristics are present in the impoverished environments where the poor live. While stress has a direct effect on illness, the second psychosocial factor, coping, has been found to moderate the stress-illness relationship. Several studies offer empirical verification that effective behavioral coping can prevent stress-induced pathology (Anisman, Pizzino, & Sklar, 1980).

While it is true that effective coping can serve as a protective factor when under stress, the social conditions under which poor people live afford little access to successful coping experiences. Mirowsky and Ross (1980) maintain that poor people are exposed to experiences that lead to a sense of powerlessness. Kessler and Cleary (1980) propose that feelings of self worth and control over the environment are positively correlated with socioeconomic status. Thus coping resources are differentially available to person of varying social positions. Poor people, who have greater exposure to stressful life events, have less access to coping resources, whether social or psychological. It is important to discover ways for providing women and disadvantaged people greater access to coping resources. One useful concept is hardiness, which is a multifaceted personality construct, consisting of a sense of control, commitment to self and to work, and of feeling challenged when confronted with change (Huang, 1995).

Theory suggests that personality hardiness moderates the stress-illness relationship through its effects on the cognitive appraisal of events as threatening and on adaptive coping. Hardiness increases the probability that events will be perceived as less threatening. Hardiness also facilitates adaptive coping or inhibits maladaptive coping (Cohen & Edwards, 1989). Theoretically, persons with high scores on hardiness use active and optimistic coping styles, which facilitate the taking of decisive actions to resolve problems (Kobasa, 1982).

Several studies have documented the relationship between stress, hardiness, and subsequent health (e.g., Hull, Van Treuren, & Virnelli, 1987; Kobasa, 1982). However, the results for buffering effects in women have been less consistent than those for men (McCranie, Lambert, & Lambert, 1987; Roth, Wiebe, Fillingim, & Shay, 1989; Schmied & Lawler, 1986). Whether hardiness effects generalize to women, and to lower socioeconomic status women, in particular, is an important question. To the extent that the environments of low- income women are less controllable and less responsive to active coping strategies, hardiness may not show the same moderation effects as found in middle-income male executives. To test this assertion, this research examined whether hardiness buffered the effects of stress on illness in lower socioeconomic status women. In addition, this present study investigated whether hardiness was associated with differences in the experience of community stressors and whether differences in levels of perceived community stress were associated with differences in illness reports.

METHOD

Participants and Data Collection

One hundred women (50 European-Americans and 50 African-Americans) with family incomes at or below the poverty line, as established by the Department of Health and Human Services of the United States Government, participated in the study. The mean age of the women was 34.1 years. The data were collected in the offices of four public housing projects and at two large supermarkets located in economically distressed areas. Participants were instructed that completion of the questionnaires constituted informed consent and were asked to read the instructions printed on each inventory before beginning to complete it. Following completion of the questionnaire packet, each individual was given a lottery ticket for a 1 in 100 chance of winning a television set,

valued at $250. The television set was awarded to one of the partici-
pants based on a random drawing of one ticket.

Measures

Socioeconomic status. Socioeconomic status was operationally defined as income level. The established yearly family income levels for
poverty ranged from $7,890 for a family of one to $27,650 for a family
of eight (1998 *Federal Register*).

Hardiness. Hardiness is a configuration of personality characteristics
operating together to strengthen resistance to the harmful effects of
stress (Kobasa, Maddi, & Kahn, 1982). It is a multifaceted personality
construct composed of control, commitment, and challenge. Control is
a belief in personal influence over the events in one's life. Commitment
is the tendency to invest oneself in the activities and events experienced
in life, thereby mitigating encounters with stressful life events. Challenge is an appreciation of the positive aspects of change, which is
viewed as stimulating and growth producing. Challenge facilitates the
effective appraisal of the threat of events.

The hardiness measure (Dispositional Resilience scale) utilized in
this current study was used in the Bartone et al. (1989) study of the influence of hardiness on health among persons who had assisted with a
military air disaster. The Dispositional Resilience scale is a 45 item,
Likert-type, modified version of a scale originally used with blue-collar
workers, and it is highly correlated with Kobasa's (1979) Unabridged
Hardiness scale (Bartone et al., 1989). The measure corrects many of
the measurement problems of the Unabridged Hardiness scale. The 45
items comprising the scale were selected on the basis of high item-scale
correlation among bus drivers (Bartone et al., 1989). Cronbach's alpha
for this measure is .85. The responses on the Dispositional Resilience
scale range from "Not at all true" (score = 0) to "Completely true"
(score = 3). Examples of the items on the instrument include "Most of
my life gets spent doing things that are worthwhile," "No matter how
hard I try, my efforts usually accomplish nothing," and "I don't like to
make changes in my every day schedule." Reliability and validity data
of the Unabridged Hardiness Scale is summarized in Kobasa, Maddi,
Pucetti, and Zola (1985). In addition, Hull, Van Treuren, and Virnelli
(1987) conducted an extensive investigation into the convergent and
discriminant validity of both the long version (Unabridged Hardiness
scale) and the short version of the hardiness measure. In several instances, the results of Hull, Van Treuren, and Virnelli's study showed

statistically significant correlations between the two forms of hardiness measures and existing measures of personality characteristics. The results showed a positive correlation between the short version measure of composite hardiness and a measure of overgeneralization ($r = .34, p < .01$). Two subscales of the hardiness measure also were correlated with overgeneralization: the commitment ($r = .21, p < .05$) and the control subscales ($r = .31, p < .01$). In a second sample included in the Hull, Van Treuren, and Virnelli study, the short form measure of hardiness was correlated with a Shyness scale. General hardiness, in this instance, was correlated with shyness ($r = .29, p < .01$), and so were two subscales: commitment ($r = .25, p < .01$) and control ($r = .26, p < .01$). The Unabridged Hardiness scale, the long version hardiness measure, was found to have a positive correlation with measures of other personality qualities. A positive correlation between hardiness and the Public subscale of Self-Consciousness was found ($r = .28, p < .01$). The Public subscale also was correlated with the hardiness subscales of Commitment ($r = .26, p < .01$) and Control ($r = .24, p < .01$). In several instances, the results showed that hardiness measures either were not correlated with certain other measures of different personality variables or were negatively correlated with such personality characteristics. The short form of the hardiness measure had a negative correlation with the Sociability scale, where both general hardiness ($r = -.17, p < .05$) and one of the subscales, Commitment, had negative correlations ($r = -.32, p < .01$).

The correlations of the hardiness measures with the Beck Depression Inventory differed across three of the samples included in the Hull, Van Treuren, and Virnelli study (1987). For the short version of the hardiness measure, composite hardiness was positively associated with the Beck Depression Inventory ($r = .45, p < .01$) in sample 1, in sample 2 ($r = .24, p < .01$), and in sample 3 ($r = .26, p < .01$). The results for the subscales of the Hardiness measure showed positive correlations for sample 1 for Commitment ($r = .39, p < .01$) and Control ($r = .44, p < .01$). Samples 2 and 3 had similar results: Commitment ($r = .24, p < .01$ and $r = .36, p < .01$, respectively) and Control ($r = .21, p < .01$, sample 3 only). The Unabridged Hardiness scale had similar results relative to the Beck Depression Inventory. For example, in sample 1, the correlation between the two measures was .45.

In addition to examining the convergent validity of the hardiness measures, Hull, Van Treuren, and Virnelli (1987) were interested in evidence of the measures discriminant validity. The results indicated no

TABLE 1. Intercorrelations Between Composite Hardiness and Its Subscales

	1	2	3	4
1. Hardiness	--	.61**	.90**	.87**
2. Challenge		--	.37**	.34**
3. Commitment			--	.70**
4. Control				--

*p < .05
**p < .01

statistically significant association between the hardiness measures and unrelated variables, including the Self-Criticism scale, the Situational Humor response Questionnaire, the Jenkins Activity Survey, and the two subscales of the Scholastic Aptitude Test. Concerns over measuring hardiness as a unitary construct have been reported in the literature by several different authors. The primary issue relates to the Challenge subscale of the hardiness measure. Consistently, the Challenge dimension behaves differently from composite hardiness and the Commitment and Control subscales. In the Hull, Van Treuren, and Virnelli study, the results for the Challenge subscale differed from those of the other measures. The Challenge subscale either had very low correlations or was not correlated with other personality measures.

The intercorrelations of the hardiness scale and its components computed for this present study are reported in Table 1. We found strong correlations between the subscales and composite hardiness, except in the instance of the challenge subscale. The correlation of the challenge subscale with the commitment and control subscales is low ($r = .37, p < .01$ and $r = .34, p < .01$, respectively). Similarly, Hull, Van Treuren, and Virnelli (1987) found relatively strong correlations between the long and short versions of the Hardiness scale ($r = .76, p < .001$) and the commitment and control subscales ($rs = .94$ and $.84$, respectively). The correlation for the challenge subscale was unacceptably low ($r = .37$).

The Unabridged Hardiness scale (long version) has received the greatest criticism and scrutiny relative to validity issues. Additional validity data has been reported by Funk and Houston (1987). These researchers reported statistically significant correlations between the long version hardiness scale and the College Maladjustment scale, $r(118) = -.40, p < .01$.

The results of the assessment of the test-retest reliability of the long and short versions of hardiness and the subscales (Hull, Van Treuren, & Virnelli, 1987) indicate highly significant correlations, with the subscale of commitment having the best test-retest correlations: short version, r(67) = .79; long version, r(63) = .90. The reliability of composite hardiness was long version, r(48) = .89; short version, r(59) = .74.

Stress. The Social Readjustment Rating scale (Holmes & Rahe, 1967) was used to measure stress level over the past 12 months. This scale contains 43 weighted items. Minor modifications were made to the scale to remove items not relevant for this sample. The deleted items were, "wife beginning or ceasing work outside the home," "change in sleeping habits," "changes in eating habits," and "personal illness." This scale has been used in the majority of the research on hardiness (e.g., Kobasa, 1979).

Illness. The illness score was the weighted sum of 126 items on the Seriousness of Illness Rating scale (Wyler, Masuda, & Holmes, 1968), completed for the past 12 months. This measure is a self-report check-list of diseases, which are weighted on the basis of prognosis, duration, threat to life, degree of disability, and degree of discomfort. Sample items from the scale are peptic ulcer with a weight of 500, sinus infection weighted 150, and heart attack with a weight of 855.

Community stress. Three scales, Fear, Social Problem, and Violence, (Cohen et al., 1982) comprised the community stress measure. The Fear subscale contains 5 items, with responses ranging from "not at all like it is" (score = 1) to "exactly like it is" (score = 4). Sample items from this subscale include "In this area, many people I know are afraid to go out at night," and "This neighborhood is really a safe place to live." In the first item, the word "many" was deleted, and in the second item the word "really" was deleted in order to moderate the extremes. The reliability coefficient for this subscale is .88. The Social Problem subscale has 6 items. The responses for this subscale range from "not a problem at all" to "very serious problem." Sample items from the subscale include "drug addicts in the neighborhood," "unemployment," and "crazy people in the streets." The reliability coefficient for this subscale is .82. The Violent Crimes subscale contains 5 items. The responses range from "never" (score = 1) to "frequently" (score = 4). Sample items from this subscale include "Someone murdered," "People being hit by the police," and "Violent arguments between neighbors." The reliability coefficient for this subscale is .78 (Cohen et al., 1982). All of the scales used a five-point Likert scale.

Demographics. Demographic information was collected on marital history, age, employment status, family composition and size, health practices, education, and income.

RESULTS

Sample Characteristics

Table 2 displays the demographic data for African-American and European-American participants in the study. The two races were similar on almost all variables. However, African-American low-income women were less likely to be unemployed (32% vs. 67.9%) and to have attended college (43.3% vs. 57.7%). Euro-American women were more likely to be divorced (82.4% vs. 17.6%), while African-American women constituted more of the Never Married (64% vs. 35.3%) category. Table 3 reports the mean scores by race for stress, illness, and hardiness. A MANOVA comparison of race indicated that there were few differences between races, with only a trend towards a race main effect ($p < .085$). Tests of the between-subjects effects indicated higher scores on the experience of violence stress ($p < .002$) and lower scores on the Challenge subscale of the Hardiness scale ($p < .01$) for the African-American women.

Hardiness Moderation Effects in Lower Socioeconomic Status Women

The first research question addressed the moderation of the stress-illness relationship by hardiness. The mean life-event stress score for the total group was 283.5, $SD = 154.08$. Life-event stress scores, in the present study, ranged from 40 to 762. The mean illness score for the total group was 2420.98, with a standard deviation of 1661.4. Simple correlations revealed a strong, positive correlation between stress and illness ($r = .487, p < .01$) and a negative correlation between hardiness and illness ($r = -.234, p = .031$). Individuals with lower scores on the hardiness scale had higher illness scores than did individuals with high scores on hardiness.

The buffering effect of hardiness was determined using hierarchical regression, entering first stress, then hardiness, stress × hardiness, race, race × stress, and stress × race × hardiness with illness as the predictor variable. As shown in Table 4, the total model was significant (multiple $R = .63, p < .01$), with 37.6% of the variance in illness scores accounted for by three factors: stress, hardiness × stress, and race × stress. In an attempt to understand the interactions of hardiness and race with stress, median split groups were used to compare illness scores for high and low

TABLE 2. Sample Characteristics

Variables	Number EA (%)[a]	Number AA (%)	Total
High school	30 (53.6)	26 (46.4)	52
Junior college	5 (27.8)	13 (72.2)	18
College	15 (57.7)	11 (42.3)	26
Unemployed	19 (67.9)	9 (32.1)	28
Employed	31 (43.7)	40 (56.3)	71
Never Married	12 (35.3)	22 (64)	34
Married	12 (50)	12 (50)	24
Divorced	14 (82.4)	3 (17.6)	17
Separated	8 (47.1)	9 (52.9)	17
Less than $8,050	17 (43.6)	22 (56.4)	39
$8,050-$22,049	22 (46.8)	25 (53.2)	47
$22,050-$27,650	6 (75)	2 (25)	8
Family size	3.64		
Age	33.65		

[a]EA = European-American, AA = African-American

groups on hardiness, stress, and race. The means for the groups are shown in Table 5. Consistent with hardiness theory, illness scores were similar for high and low hardiness women under conditions of low stress, but under high levels of stress, illness scores were reduced for women with higher scores on hardiness. Similarly, Euro-American and African-American women have comparable illness scores at low levels of stress, but at higher levels of stress, being African-American protects against stress-related increases in illness. Thus, in this sample, two stress buffers emerged, being hardy and being African-American.

Association of Hardiness with Differences in Levels of Community Stress

Whether differences in the experience of community stressors were associated with personality hardiness and whether these differences were associated with illness are additional questions examined in this study. T-tests, comparing the group mean scores of low and high hardy low SES women, were performed in order to establish whether these two groups differed in their scores on community stress. The group mean community stress score, for women with low scores on hardiness, was 35, with a standard deviation of 9.27 compared with a group mean score of 26.5, with a standard deviation of 9, for women who scored high on hardiness. The results from t-tests indicated a significant difference between the means of the two groups, $t(79) = 4.155$, $p < .0001$. Women with low hardiness scores reported higher levels of community

TABLE 3. Race Comparisons on Stress, Illness, and Personality Hardiness

Measures	EA Mean (SE)[b]		AA Mean	
Life event stress[a]	275.7	(22.1)	291.4	(21.7)
Community stress	29.2	(1.35)	33.0	(1.61)
Fear scale	9.5	(.43)	9.8	(.54)
Social problem scale	11.9	(.91)	12.9	(.88)
Violence scale	7.7	(.42)	10.4	(.58)
Illness	2663.2	(262.6)	2183.6	(198.0)
Hardiness	83.0	(.04)	79.0	(.05)
Challenge scale	22.2	(.04)	20.4	(.04)
Commitment scale	30.7	(.07)	29.0	(.07)
Control scale	30.1	(.05)	28.5	(.07)

[a]Alpha coefficients for these scales, based on the current sample, were Stress (.73), Fear (.73), Social problems (.96), Violence (.82), Illness (.78), Hardiness (.80).
[b]EA = European-American, AA = African-American, N = 50 for each race

TABLE 4. Hierarchical Regression Analysis of Hardiness as a Predictor of Illness

Measure	R	r^2	Beta
Stress	.486***	.236	2.1
Hardiness	.575	.26	.17
Race	.554	.31	.13
Hardiness × Stress	.593**	.35	−1.16
Race × Stress	.621*	.39	−.69
Hardiness × Stress × Race	.625	.39	.66

***$p < .0001$
**$p < .016$
*$p < .025$

stress, in general, and higher levels on all three of the subscales (fear, social problems, and violence).

Stress, as traditionally measured by the Holmes and Rahe (1967) check-list, was found to be related to illness on its own ($r = 49$, $p < .0001$). It was of interest to determine whether community stress was predictive of illness, also. Correlations were computed between illness and community stress, with no significant results obtained. Thus, while hardy women may perceive their neighborhoods as less stressful rela-

TABLE 5. Illness (SE) for Hardiness, Stress, and Race Groups

	Low Stress	n	High Stress	n
Low Hardiness	1839.4 (295.5)	23	3281.4 (395.3)	27
High Hardiness	1870.4 (224.8)	27	2633.9 (295.4)	23
European-American	1951.8 (245.5)	28	3552.5 (445.6)	22
African-American	1734.4 (269.4)	22	2536.6 (268.7)	28

tive to violence, social problems, and fear, this appraisal of the neighborhood does not relate directly to decreased illness.

DISCUSSION

The purpose of this research was to determine the role of personality hardiness in buffering the stress-illness relationship in women living in poverty. Consistent with the theoretical basis of hardiness and with empirical results obtained by Kobasa and colleagues (1982), highly stressed, lower socioeconomic status women, who were high on personality hardiness, were less compromised by stressful life events than were low hardiness women. Furthermore, this effect was not moderated by race; hardiness was beneficial to both African-American and European-American women. Both hardiness and race moderate the stress-illness relationship, with high hardy and African-American women being healthier, when experiencing stress, than their low hardy and European-American counterparts. When levels of stress were low, hardiness and racial groups did not differ. There were few differences between races to explain the lower stress-related illness levels of African-American women.

Because poor people often live in communities where they are exposed to conditions very different from those of the communities where higher socioeconomic status persons live, this research examined community stress. Community stress has been found to be associated with feeling bad. It also is negatively correlated with feelings of well-being. In contrast, in this sample, community stress was not associated with illness. However, it was linked to hardiness. High hardy women reported less community stress than did women with low scores on hardiness. Since all of the women in this sample lived in the same general area, this suggests that high hardy, lower socioeconomic women may perceive their communities as less threatening and overwhelming. This is consistent with hardiness theory, which proposes that hardiness facilitates the accurate perception of events, rendering them as less threatening. Further research should explore the bases of this differential perception.

Study Limitations

There are two limitations of this study that need mentioning. First, we assessed only physical illness over the past year and not psychological distress. Stress and hardiness may impact psychological health as well, but hardiness buffering effects relative to the stress-distress relationship cannot be determined from these data. Secondly, these results are derived from concurrent measures of stress, hardiness, and illness. To the extent that sick individuals feel more stressed, less hardy, and more passive, no causal inference can be drawn. However, the majority of the early studies on stress and illness also were concomitant, and this study validates the generalization of those results to African-American and Caucasian, lower socioeconomic women. Given that this population often has higher levels of illness than the general population, more attention should be paid to the determinants of health in this group. Ideally, future studies would employ a longitudinal design and would examine rural and urban dwellers. Additionally, future studies should examine the general population of both male and female African-Americans.

Implications for Practice

The results from this study indicate that hardiness reduced the severity of illness experienced by lower income women who were challenged with highly stressful situations. In addition, poor women with hardy personality characteristics perceived their neighborhoods as less threatening. These beneficial effects of the hardy personality indicate the need to increase opportunities for involvement in experiences that foster a sense of commitment, control, and challenge. Persons with hardy personality qualities believe that they have personal influence over the events in their lives, a quality Kobasa (1979) labeled "control," which some researchers consider a critical determinant of stress induced pathologies (Anisman, Pizzino, & Sklar, 1980). These researchers found evidence that exposure to uncontrollable stressors results in increased ulceration and enhanced both development and growth of tumors. The literature provides ample evidence of the importance of psychosocial variables in illness. The results from the present study, strengthened by the stress and hardiness literature, provide support for the importance of interventions directed to empowering individuals and to increasing a sense of competence and mastery in dealing with stressful life situations, in meeting environmental challenges, and in making full use of environmental resources (Kemp, Whittaker, & Tracy, 1997).

Practice approaches that emphasize a strengths perspective offer greater opportunities for increasing an individual's sense of control, challenge, and commitment. Opportunities for experiencing the self as a capable and competent organism foster the growth of personality hardiness. A practice informed by the values of the person's right to self-determination and individualization engenders such opportunities. Strength-based practice involves individuals in each aspect of treatment and keeps them informed about the intervention process. This means that practitioners must recast helping relationships as collaborative partnerships and select empowerment-based practice orientations.

The findings of this study also indicate those lower socioeconomic status women with higher scores on the hardiness scales, perceived their environments as less threatening than did women without these personality characteristics. These results are consistent with the understanding that there are multiple realities, which are mediated by individual systems of meaning. They support the growing interest in the social construction of reality, including the use of narrative and story as elements of practice (Kemp, Whittaker, & Tracy, 1997).

Implications for Policy

The contemporary political climate of devolution (Nathan, 1995), diminishing federal responsibility, and cost-containment policies will present challenges for offering to lower socioeconomic status women expanded opportunities for self-determination and participation in decision-making processes. Indeed these ideals seem hardly attainable in this era of federal and state funding cuts, and major philosophical shifts in the premises underlying social policy (Kamerman, 1996).

Suggestions that the present political climate, absent the influence of the Social Work profession, promises to return the United States to an era of restraint and punishment, reflective of 17th century England and colonial America, or to a time when there was no federal responsibility for individual citizens are emerging. Freeman (1996) suggests that contemporary policymakers' biased definitions of self-sufficiency and related social program reforms encourage punitive policies. The Newt Gingrich and Dick Armey *Contract with America* has rekindled the ongoing debate over the role of government in public welfare. The Contract with America returns us to the pre depression era of limited federal government responsibility and to a time of blaming individuals for their stations in life rather than examining the influences of macro social structures. Current social welfare policies revive old Calvinistic views of poor people (Dolgoff, Feldstein, & Skolnik, 1997, p. 8). These Calvinistic views are antithetical to the development of personality hardiness, which is characterized by adaptive coping and self-efficacy. With this in mind, more ought to be done to ensure that the consumers of social welfare participate in decision-making at critical points in the process, and policymakers must not overlook the importance of personal choice and belief in one's personal competence as they work at revolutionizing social welfare policies.

Implications for Knowledge of Human Behavior

The findings from this study are opposite to many in the literature that show higher rates of illness in minority samples (e.g., Blendon et al., 1995; Kessler & Neighbors, 1986) and reinforce the importance of equating racial groups on SES. There were few differences between races to explain the lower stress-related illness levels of African-American women. However, it was informally observed that African-American women were more likely to utilize services offered through public housing offices, such as counseling and child care assistance. This provides support for the importance of social support systems, self-esteem, and self-efficacy for social functioning and for maintaining health.

Empirical evidence of hardiness moderator effects in African-American, low-income women is important because of the greater impact of poverty for this group. The findings from this present study offer empirical confirmation that hardiness effects extend to low SES females, who are quite different from the white, middle class executives studied in the original research. This study extends our knowledge that hardiness effects can generalize to other groups and to other contexts. However, there remains a need to better understand the contexts within which hardiness effects are important to the stress-illness relationship.

The results of this current study provide evidence that women with high scores on hardiness had lower scores on community stress, which was found to influence illness in this population of women. It is reasonable that women with high scores on hardiness appraise neighborhood occurrences like violence, drug abuse, and unsafe conditions as less threatening and overwhelming than do women with lower scores on hardiness. According to Kobasa and Puccetti (1983), the challenge disposition directs individuals to find opportunities for decision-making and to evaluate events in the context of an overall plan. For low-income women, the challenge disposition would help to reduce potential disruptions associated with stressful community events. Increases in the levels of challenge may lead to better decision-making and more adaptive cognitive appraisals, which attenuate the physiological arousal precipitated by stressful events (Funk, 1992). The environment influences coping effectiveness through shaping the appraisals and behavioral dispositions of individuals (Kessler & Cleary, 1980). Economically impoverished communities provide little social resources for coping effectively with stressful events; some theorists have posited that this lack of social resources explains why lower SES persons are more affected by stressful life events.

The hardiness literature suggests that individuals who believe in their own effectiveness take decisive action and use active rather than passive coping styles. Persons with passive coping styles rely on devices that help them tolerate stress. Alcohol and drug addiction are two examples of how people manage to forget their problems (Kessler & Cleary, 1980). The beneficial effects of hardiness on adaptive coping and cognitive appraisals suggest that identifying factors that promote the development of commitment, challenge, and a sense of self-effectiveness is important for low-socioeconomic status females who are disproportionately exposed to stressful life events. It is important to understand both how hardiness develops and how macro social structures operate to shape hardiness within the individual. Understanding hardiness as a resistance resource is a start toward gaining greater knowledge of the importance of personality factors to individual differences in illness susceptibility. Resolving the problem of why some people become ill when under stress and others do not continues to be a major barrier to understanding the stress-illness link.

REFERENCES

Anisman, H., Pizzino, A., & Sklar, L. S. (1980). Coping with stress: Norepinephrine depletion and escape performance. *Brain Research, 191,* 583-588.

Baizman, E. R., Cox, B. M., Osman, O. H., & Goldstein, A. (1979). Experimental alterations of Endorphin levels in rat pituitary. *Neuroendocrinology, 28,* 402-424.

Bartone, P. T., Ursano, R. J., Wright, K. M., & Inhraham, L. H. (1989). The impact of a military disaster on the health of assistance workers: A prospective study. *The Journal of Nervous and Mental Disease, 177,* 317-328.

Belle, D. E. (1982). The impact of poverty on social networks and supports. *Marriage and Family Review, 5* (4), 89-101.

Blendon, R. J., Scheck, A. C., Donelan, K., Hill, C. A., Smith, M., Dennis, B., & Altman, D. (1995). How whites and African Americans view their health and social problems: Different experiences, different expectations. *Journal of the American Medical Association, 273* (6), 34-44.

Cohen, S., & Edwards, J. R. (1989). Personality characteristics as moderators of the relationship between stress and disorder. In R. Neufeld (Ed.), *Advances in the Investigation of Psychological Stress* (pp. 235-283). New York: Wiley.

Cohen, P., Struening, E. L., Genevie, L. E., Kaplan, S. R., Muhlin, G. I., & Peck, H. B. (1992). Community stressors, mediating conditions and wellbeing in urban neighborhoods. *Journal of Community Psychology, 10,* 377-391.

Dohrenwend, B. S. (1973). Social status and stressful life events. *Journal of Personality and Social Psychology, 28* (2), 225-235.

Dolgoff, R., Feldstein, D., & Skolnik, L. (1997). *Understanding Social Welfare* (4th ed.). New York: Longman.

Freeman, E. M. (1996). Welfare reform and services for children and families: Setting a new practice, research, and policy agenda. *Social Work, 41* (5), 521-532.

Funk, S. C. (1992). Hardiness: A review of theory and research. *Health Psychology, 11*(5), 335-345.

Funk, S. C., & Houston, B. K. (1987). A critical analysis of the Hardiness scale's validity and utility. *Journal of Personality and Social Psychology, 53*(3), 572-578.

Holmes, T. H., & Rahe, R. H. (1967). The social readjustment rating scale. *Journal of Psychosomatic Research, 11,* 213-218.

Huang, C. (1995). Hardiness and stress: A critical review. *Maternal-Child Nursing Journal, 23* (3), 82-89.

Hull, J. G., Van Treuren, R. R., & Virnelli, S. (1987). Hardiness and health: A critique and alternative approach. *Journal of Personality and Social Psychology, 53* (3), 518-530.

Ingram, K. M., Corning, A. F., & Schmidt, L. D. (1996). The relationship of victimization experiences to psychological well-being among homeless women and low-income housed women. *Journal of Counseling Psychology, 43* (2), 218-227.

Kamerman, S. (1996). The new politics of child and family policies. *Social Work, 41*(5), 453-565.

Kaplan, R., Anderson, J., & Wingard, D. (1991). Gender differences in health-related quality of life. *Health Psychology, 10,* 86-93.

Kemp, S. P., Whittaker, J. K., & Tracy, E. M. (1997). *Person Environment Practice: The Social Ecology on Interpersonal Helping.* New York, NY: Aldine DeGruyter.

Kessler, R. C., & Cleary, P. D. (1980). Social class and psychological distress. *American Psychological Review, 45* (June), 463-478.

Kessler, R. C., & McLeod, J. D. (1984). Sex differences in vulnerability to undesirable life events. *American Sociological Review, 49* (October), 620-631.

Kessler, R. C., & McRae, J. A. (1981). Trends in the relationship between sex and psychological distress: 1957-1976. *American Sociological Review, 46,* 443-452.

Kessler, R. C., & Neighbors, H. W. (1986). A new perspective on the relationship among race, social class, and psychological distress. *Journal of Health and Social Behavior, 27, 107-115.*

Kobasa, S. C. (1979). Stressful life events, personality, and health: An inquiry into hardiness. *Journal of Personality and Social Psychology, 37,* 1-11.

Kobasa, S. C. (1982). Commitment and coping in stress resistance among lawyers. *Journal of Personality and Social Psychology, 42* (4), 707-717.

Kobasa, S. C., Maddi, S. R., & Courington, S. (1981). Personality and constitution as mediators in the stress-illness relationship. *Journal of Health and Social Behavior, 22* (December), 368-378.

Kobasa, S. C., Maddi, S. R., & Kahn, S. (1982). Hardiness and health: A prospective study. *Journal of Personality and Social Psychology, 42* (1), 168-177.

Kobasa, S. C., Maddi, S. R., Pucetti, M. C., & Zola, M. A. (1985). Effectiveness of hardiness, exercise, and social support as resources against illness. *Journal of Psychosomatic Research, 29,* 525-533.

Kobasa, S. C. O., & Pucetti, M. C. (1983). Personality and social resources in stress resistance. *Journal of Personality and Social Psychology, 45* (4), 839-850.

Kvetnansky, R., Kopin, I. J., & Saavedra, J. M. (1978). Changes in epinephrine in individual hypothalamic nuclei after immobilization stress. *Brain Research, 155,* 387-390.

Lawler, K. A., & Schmied, L. A. (1987). The relationship of stress, Type A behavior, and powerlessness to physiological responses in female clerical workers. *Journal of Psychosomatic Research, 31* (6), 555-566.

Marmot, M. G. (1994). Social differentials in health within and between populations. *Daedalus, 123* (3), 193-216.

Marmot, M. G., Shipley, M. J., & Rose, G. (1984). Inequalities in death: Specific explanations of a general pattern? *The Lancet* (May 5), 1003-1006.

McCranie, E. W., Lambert, V. A., & Lambert, C. E. (1987). Work, stress, hardiness, and burnout among hospital staff nurses. *Nursing Research, 36,* 374-378.

Mirowsky, J., & Ross, C. E. (1980). Minority status, ethnic culture, and distress: A comparison of Blacks, Whites, Mexicans, and Mexican-Americans. *American Journal of Sociology, 86,* 479-495.

Nathan, R. P. (1995). *Hard Road Ahead: Block Grants and the "Devolution Revolution."* Albany, NY: Nelson A. Rockefeller Institute of Government.

Northrop, E. M. (1990). The feminization of poverty: The demographic factor and the composition of economic growth. *Journal of Economic Issues, 24* (1), 160.

Pappas, G., Queen, S. H., Hadden, W., & Fisher, G. (1993). The increasing disparity in mortality between socioeconomic groups in the United States, 1960 and 1986. *The New England Journal of Medicine, 329* (2), 103-109, 774.

Rainwater, L. (1970). *Behind ghetto walls.* Chicago: Aldine Publishing Company.

Roth, D. L., Wiebe, D. J., Fillingim, R. B., & Shay, K. A. (1989). Life events, fitness, hardiness, and health: A simultaneous analysis of proposed stress resistance effects. *Journal of Personality and Social Psychology, 57,* 136-142.

Schmied, L. A., & Lawler, K. A. (1986). Hardiness, type A behavior, and the stress-illness relation in working women. *Journal of Personality and Social Psychology, 51* (6), 1218-1223.

Siegrist, J. (1995). Social differentials in chronic disease: What can sociological knowledge offer to explain and possibly reduce them. *Social Science Medicine, 41* (12), 1603-1605.

Thomas, S. P. (1997). Distressing aspects of women's roles, vicarious stress, and health consequences. *Issues in Mental Health Nursing, 18,* 539-557.

Wilkinson, R. G. (1992). Income distribution and life expectancy. *British Medical Journal, 304,* 165-168.

Williams, D. R. (1990). Socioeconomic differentials in health: A review and redirection. *Social Psychology Quarterly, 53* (2), 81-99.

Wyler, A. R., Masuda, M., & Holmes, T. H. (1968). Seriousness of illness rating scale. *Journal of Psychosomatic Research, 11,* 363-374.

Environmental Concern
and Personal Health Behaviors
in Women

Jill Greenwald Robbins
Shelly A. Wiechelt

SUMMARY. Effective efforts to shift attitudes and behaviors impacting the health of the ecological environment may be found to be similar to those efforts that are effective for changing personal health behaviors. This investigation examines the relationship between environmental attitudes and self-care behaviors in a sample of twenty-seven women in their forties. Environmental concern, as measured by an updated version of Weigel and Weigel's (1978) Environmental Concern Scale, was significantly correlated with self-reported personal health care behaviors as measured by a new self-report Health Questionnaire. Implications for social work practice and future research are discussed.

Jill Greenwald Robbins, PhD, is Psychologist, Salem Psychological Associates, Salem, New Hampshire.

Shelly A. Wiechelt, PhD, is Assistant Professor, School of Social Work, University at Buffalo, State University of New York.

Address correspondence to: Jill Greenwald Robbins, PhD, 87 Stiles Road, Suite 106, Salem, NH 03079 or Shelly A. Wiechelt, PhD, Assistant Professor, University at Buffalo, SUNY, 685 Baldy Hall, Buffalo, NY 14260.

The authors gratefully acknowledge the assistance of Ricky Greenwald and Philip Robbins.

This article is based on dissertation research, which was funded by an Environmental Conservation Fellowship from the National Wildlife Federation to Jill Greenwald Robbins.

[Haworth co-indexing entry note]: "Environmental Concern and Personal Health Behaviors in Women." Robbins, Jill Greenwald, and Shelly A. Wiechelt. Co-published simultaneously in *Journal of Human Behavior in the Social Environment* (The Haworth Social Work Practice Press, an imprint of The Haworth Press, Inc.) Vol. 7, No. 3/4, 2003, pp. 141-158; and: *Women and Girls in the Social Environment: Behavioral Perspectives* (ed: Nancy J. Smyth) The Haworth Social Work Practice Press, an imprint of The Haworth Press, Inc., 2003, pp. 141-158. Single or multiple copies of this article are available for a fee from The Haworth Document Delivery Service [1-800-HAWORTH, 9:00 a.m. - 5:00 p.m. (EST). E-mail address: docdelivery@haworthpress.com].

Digital Object Identifier: 10.1300/J137v7n03_09

KEYWORDS. Environmental concern, attitudes, health behaviors, women

Ecological sustainability is currently threatened (State of the World, 1999; Oskamp, 2000). Poor environmental conditions are caused primarily by human behaviors. Human behavior change, therefore, is critical to any solution. Efforts to improve environmental conditions traditionally have come from sciences such as biology, chemistry, and geology. More recently there has been increasing recognition that the social and behavioral sciences must play a central role in these important interdisciplinary efforts, since social and behavioral sciences offer means of understanding and changing human attitudes and behaviors (Howard, 2000; McKenzie-Mohr, 2000; Oskamp, 2000; Stern, 2000; Winter, 2000).

The social work literature emphasizes the promotion of approaching human problems in terms of the person-in-environment. The ecological perspective of social work (Germain & Gitterman, 1996) provides a framework for understanding and impacting human problems in the context of the person in his or her social and physical environments. The physical environments include both the built and natural world. The reciprocal relationship that exists between people and the environment suggests that failure to care for either the person or the environment will result in damage to both the person and the environment. Thus, social work brings the perspective that adaptation on the part of humans to achieve "goodness-of-fit" with the environment is paramount. It is important, then, to increase our understanding of the factors that obstruct or promote attitudes and behaviors consistent with such adaptation.

Social and psychological studies have looked at environmental attitudes and behaviors by relating environmental attitudes and actions to broader belief systems (Dunlap & Van Liere, 1984), to adult developmental positions (Robbins & Greenwald 1994), to worldviews, such as one favoring "egalitarian rather than hierarchical or individualistic social relationships" (Dake, 1992, cited in Winter, 2000), and to gender (Wilson, Daly, Gordon, & Pratt, 1996), among others. Researchers have examined the impact (or lack thereof) on behavior change of educational efforts (McKenzie-Mohr, 2000), of changing situational factors

(Gardner & Stern, 1996), and of contingency management (Walker, 1979), among other factors. This growing body of research, which has looked directly at the relevance of psychological theories to environmental attitudes and behaviors, is important to the effort toward sustainability.

Outside of the environmental literature may be another rich source of potentially relevant findings. In particular, much of the health psychology literature could be relevant to the environmental realm. There are two reasons for this premise. First, health psychology typically tackles problems with much in common with those being explored in the environmental area. Note the similarities as Miller, Shoda, and Hurley (1996) speak of health psychology:

> There has been an explosion of interest and research in health psychology in the last decade, fueled by the excitement of successfully applying basic psychological concepts to understand how people deal with health challenges (e.g., Baum & Singer, 1987; Gatchel, Baum, & Krantz, 1989; Lazarus, 1991; Leventhal, 1983; Rodin & Salovey, 1989; Weiss, 1992). This rapidly growing field encompasses disease prevention and early detection, as well as short- and long-term management of disease course and consequences (Taylor, 1990, 1995). It is also concerned with individual differences in selecting and processing information about health-related risks, needs, and stressors.

As is apparent, the challenges tackled by the health psychology literature are similar to those being tackled by those trying to improve environmentally related behavior. In each, one must address at an individual and societal level such topics as education, prevention, compliance, and perception of short- and long-term risk and gain, where the risks of certain types of action or inaction can be quite severe.

A second reason for the premise that it could be useful to study environmental behaviors in relation to health behaviors is that directly or indirectly, environmental behaviors *are* health behaviors. Our personal health depends upon the health of the wider environment, and choices about one may have an impact upon the other. A person choosing to use non-toxic pest control is avoiding personal exposure to materials that could hold health risks, while simultaneously protecting the environment from toxic compounds. Similarly, a hole in the ozone layer, caused largely by human behavior, leads to skin cancer. It would be logical for there to be a relationship between health behaviors and environmental concern. The former entails caring directly for the self. The latter entails caring indirectly about the self through the environment in which the self must live, and upon which the self depends.

We certainly cannot assume the existence of specific connections between particular health behaviors and particular environmental behaviors. Yet it might be useful for the sake of further illustrating the concept of a health/environment relationship to imagine specific connections, whereby people concerned about personal health issues similarly might be concerned about environmental health issues. For example, it would not be difficult to imagine a group of non-smokers being more upset by increased air pollution than a group of smokers. In each case, a person is tolerant, or not, of polluted air going into his or her body. One might imagine a person who exercises his or her body regularly being someone who would care about clean drinking water. And perhaps someone who always wears a seatbelt would apply his or her health preventive orientation even for low incidence events to an appraisal of the importance of double barrels on oil tankers for extra spill protection. Although the oil spill risk is once removed from a person's immediate health, it does still contribute to the health risk inherent in environmental degradation.

If a connection between these two fields holds up empirically, it may be fruitful for each field to be informed by the literature of the other. We have a body of research on personal health and safety attitudes and behaviors, which perhaps also could be usefully examined in relation to environmental health and safety. For example, Lindsay and Strathman (1997) took the Health Belief Model (HBM) (Rosenstock, 1990; Rosenstock & Kirscht, 1974, cited in Lindsay and Strathman, 1997) which has been found to predict health behaviors (Janz & Becker, 1984), modified it, and successfully applied it in the environmental realm. They found that the traditional and modified versions of the HBM significantly predicted recycling behavior. In the HBM, health behaviors were thought to be a function of beliefs about the following four factors: "the likelihood of a negative event, the severity of the event, the benefits associated with a certain preventive action, and the costs associated with performing that action" (p. 1803). It makes sense that these beliefs about perceived threat and outcome expectancy, which had been found predictive of health behaviors, would be relevant for environmental behaviors as well.

Looking at the two literatures, one can discover parallel findings even where studies have not connected the two fields. For example, Stern (2000) and Stern, Young, and Drickman (1992) speak of the necessity of structural interventions for affecting environmental behaviors, just as Cohen, Scribner, and Farley (2000) call for structural interventions for prevention and reduction of high-risk health behaviors. The four health behavior categories they identify are: "(1) availability of protective or harmful consumer products, (2) physical structures (or physical characteristics of products), (3) social structures and policies, and (4) media and cultural messages." Perhaps, then, effective efforts to make exercising more widely regularly practiced would have some parallels to effective efforts to make recycling more widely regularly practiced. In each, a behavior change effort might include providing easy products or structures (inexpensive, readily available, easy to use home exercise equipment; curbside pick-up), incentive programs/policies (insurance rates reduced with health club membership; a per/bag fee imposed for non-recycled garbage), and a media campaign to help make such behaviors normative.

One specific area of health research that could be of particular interest to those studying environmental behavior change is that which examines efforts to increase the use of mammography and cervical examinations. Obtaining gynecological examinations and mammograms entails a willingness to make an active effort to discover an otherwise imperceptible (at the time) long-term danger to the self (cervical or breast cancer). There are striking parallels with what is entailed in addressing possible long-term environmental health risks. This, too, requires a willingness to take action to discover otherwise imperceptible damage (e.g., depletion of the ozone layer, or a build-up of carcinogens in the ground water) before it has become too great. In each case, the inquiring individual (or company or government) knows before inquiring that unpleasant results could demand unpleasant, expensive, and possibly time-consuming efforts at treatment, which may not even be successful, especially if detection was late. Actions needed to detect personal and environmental health problems are commonly avoided.

There are many people who do face and act responsibly with health and environmental issues. Although there are many reasons to believe that the issues of personal and environmental health are related, the question remains: Are people who actively take care of their bodies in fact more likely than those who do not to be concerned about environmental issues? Or, similarly, are those who are aware of and concerned about environmental issues more likely than those who are not to take actions to protect their bodies? This study is an initial investigation into the question of whether concern for the external environment, including self-report that one would behave in an environmentally caring manner, corresponds to a positive treatment of one's own internal environment–that is, through personal, physical health related behaviors. It was expected that there would be a positive relationship between health behaviors and environmental concern.

The focus of this initial study was on women. Although much of the human impact on the environment comes from decisions made in politics, industry, and business (Stern, 2000), where men continue to be dominant, women are rapidly increasing their influence in these domains. Additionally, women continue to be the primary shoppers, as well as the primary educators in this culture. As such, women collectively can have a strong impact on environmental quality. Also, women at times have joined forces effectively to change behaviors and norms that negatively impact the family and community, such as through the temperance movement, and more recently through efforts such as Mothers Against Drunk Drivers (MADD). The role of women in the change process is an important one. Additionally, understanding the relationship between environmental concern and health behaviors for women may provide insight into focal points for preventive and interventive efforts to address what may be a synergistic relationship between care for the environment and care for the self. The knowledge gained may be useful in engaging women in a change process that could impact social attitudes, human health, and environmental concerns.

METHOD

Procedure

A sample of 27 American-born women in their forties was randomly selected from a street list of women in their forties in Greenfield, Massachusetts. Women in this age group were identified for participation in the study because they are likely to have solidified attitudes by middle-age, mid-life is often a period of increased generativity, and the need for mammography begins.

The current study was conducted as an aspect of a larger study examining environmental attitudes in depth, for which the geographical location and nationality of participants were limited, and in which participants were involved in two sessions of extensive one-on-one interviews and other measures. The measures presented in this paper were administered on the first day, following a lengthy interview about ways in which the women think about the environment. At the conclusion of the first day, participants were paid $5.00. The study was conducted in conference rooms of relatively neutral sites in the town of Greenfield. Two participants were interviewed at their homes (one did not drive and one was disabled).

Each potential participant received a letter of introduction and intent 1 to 7 days prior to being contacted by telephone for scheduling. Both the letter and the phone call emphasized the study's focus on understanding *all different ways* people think about the environment. In total, 77 names were selected. Two of the listings did not match any listing in the telephone book and were therefore not contacted. Seventy-five letters were mailed. Out of the 75 women contacted, 33 women said yes, 34 said no, 4 had moved and 4 others were not reached. Most of the women who said no indicated that they did not have the time. Some referred to illness or recent death in the family. A few would state only that they were not interested. Of those who were not reached, one repeatedly did not answer her telephone, and three with unpublished numbers did not respond to a follow-up invitational note. Of those who agreed to participate, four women were unable to attend within the needed time frame, and one had to drop out due to medical complications. Twenty-eight women participated in the study. All 28 completed the study in full. One, however, was not included in the analysis, since she was from another country. This left 27 participants. All were white. On other socio-demographic variables, there was a wide range.

Measures

Health Questionnaire. A brief self-report scale to measure personal health behaviors was developed by one of the authors (Greenwald, 1992). The measure was designed to gather data on the frequency of personal behaviors commonly considered to be positively or negatively related to short- and long-term physical health. These behaviors were smoking cigarettes, drinking alcoholic beverages, exercising, wearing a seatbelt, and obtaining mammograms and gynecological/physical examinations. The seven questions on the health questionnaire were analyzed according to the five behaviors represented (see Appendix). The two alcohol consumption questions were combined by multiplying drinking-days-per-week by drinks-per-day-when-drinking, resulting in a number representing drinks per week. The gynecological/physical examination and mammogram responses were combined by using the mean score of the two answers. In an effort to try to achieve face validity, efforts were made to have comparable scores in the five categories have roughly comparable health significance (see Appendix). The scores for the five items were summed to obtain a total score, with higher scores reflected healthier behaviors. The highest possible score was 20. Inter-item correlations based on standardized scores correlating each item to all other items excluding the item itself ranged from .11 to .42. Full-scale inter-item correlations based on standardized scores ranged from .45 to .69. The alpha coefficient was .46 based on raw ratings and .45 based on standardized scores.

Environmental Concern Scale (ECS). For a standardized, commonly used measure of beliefs and feelings about the environment, Weigel and Weigel's (1978) Environmental Concern Scale was administered. The ECS was developed in New England towns and tested in Eastern and Western towns and cities of the United States. Each community sampled had a population of fewer than 100,000. The samples had socio-economic, but limited ethnic, diversity. Each of these factors is consistent with the conditions of the proposed study. The ECS has been satisfactorily tested for internal consistency, test-retest reliability, and validity. Weigel and Weigel obtained an internal consistency alpha co-efficient of .85 and a homogeneity ratio of .26 over the six-year interval during which the surveys were conducted. The test-retest correlation obtained with a six-week interval was .83. The scale was tested for validity with a known-groups comparison test contrasting scores of randomly sampled adults with Sierra Club members. As expected, the mean concern score was higher ($p < .02$) and the standard deviation smaller with the Sierra Club members ($M = 54.5$, $SD = 6.6$) than with the other adults ($M = 44.2$, $SD = 8.4$). The significance of this difference was measured with a sign test finding the scale scores of the Sierra Club members significantly greater ($X^2 = 77.32$, $p < .001$). In addition, the scale's measurement of attitudinal differences was able to account for 38% of the variance of environmentally oriented behaviors measured in three long-term studies conducted by Weigel and Weigel.

The ECS consists of sixteen items on a range of pollution and conservation issues. Nine of the items are negatively stated, such as "Pollution is not personally affecting my life." Seven are positively stated, such as "I'd be willing to make personal sacrifices for the sake of slowing down pollution even though the immediate results may not seem significant." The participants were asked to rate each statement on a five-point scale ranging from "strongly agree" to "strongly disagree."

Two of the sixteen items of the original ECS were outdated and therefore replaced, on the suggestion of the primary author of the original scale. Item #2, which originally read "We should not worry about killing too many game animals because in the long run things will balance out," was replaced with "We should not worry about filling too many wetlands since there are so many of them." Item #11, which was originally "Predators such as hawks, crows, skunks, and coyotes which prey on farmers' grain crops and poultry should be eliminated," was replaced with "Insects which destroy farmers' crops should be eliminated, with as much pesticide as it takes." In addition, the wording of #5 was changed slightly. Instead of "The benefits of modern consumer products are more important than the pollution that results from their production and use," the statement now reads, "The benefits of modern consumer products are more important than the environmental problems that result from their production and use." With this small word substitution, the current problems of ozone depletion and global warming are more readily included.

Items were analyzed according to the questionnaire's scale, reversing scores on those items that were oriented in a negative direction. That is, high scores were always indicative of environmentally concerned responses, regardless of the wording of the question. Item analysis of the original 14 questions revealed that two of the questions (numbers 5 and 14) that correlated well in Weigel's samples did not in the current sample. They correlated with the remaining 12 questions at .11 and .06 respectively. By Weigel's recommendation, these two items were therefore excluded from the remaining analyses. The two replacement questions (numbers 2 and 11) correlated well with the other 12 questions, at .42 and .45 respectively, and were therefore included for the remaining analyses. The alpha coefficient for the final scale was .75 based on the raw ratings, and .78 based on those scores transformed to standardized scores.

The Health Questionnaire and the Environmental Concern Scale were analyzed together to determine whether personal (internal) health behaviors as indicated by this self-report scale are correlated with concern about the health of the (external) environment, as indicated by the ECS.

RESULTS

Health Behaviors

Although participants were instructed that they need not respond to anything that may make them uncomfortable, all of the women responded to all of the questions. With the exception that no one reported consuming more than eight drinks per week, each scoring category was represented across its full range. The mean score (with 4 representing the most healthful possible response in each category) for drinks was 3.52 ($SD = 0.58$), for cigarettes was 3.52 ($SD = 1.05$), for exercise was 3.22 ($SD = 0.85$), for seatbelt use was 3.19 ($SD = 0.92$), and for gynecological/physical exam or mammogram was 3.35 ($SD = 0.89$). The total mean score was 16.80 ($SD = 2.45$) out of a possible total of 20.

Environmental Concern

The women in this study scored quite high on the ECS. Even the least environmentally aware participant responded in extremes, receiving close to the highest possible concern score: On a five-point scale, the (adjusted for positive or negative wording) item means ranged from 3.5 to 4.5, with the SDs ranging from .51 to 1.14, resulting in a total mean score of 57.7 ($SD = 5.9$). Adjusting that score to correspond with the scoring of Weigel's original samples (two more questions and a Likert scale from 0-4 rather than from 1-5) resulted in an adjusted mean of 52.7 ($SD = 5.4$). In comparison, Weigel's 1974-1976 randomly selected Eastern sample had a mean score of only 44.2 ($SD = 8.4$). His Sierra Club (i.e., more likely to be concerned) sample averaged 54.5 ($SD = 6.6$).

Relationship Between Health Behavior and Environmental Concern

There was a statistically significant positive correlation of .40 (using Z-Scores: $F(1, 25) = 4.87$, $p < .05$) between environmental concern as measured by the adjusted version of the ECS, and self-reported health related behaviors generally associated with the care a woman takes of herself as measured by the HQ. These results indicate that there may be a moderately strong relationship between personal health behaviors and environmental concern.

DISCUSSION

Relationship Between Health Behaviors and Environmental Concern

The results of this preliminary study indicate a positive relationship between self-reported environmental concern, and health preventive and health non-destructive behaviors. The fact that significant results were obtained despite a small sample size and a narrow range of scores on both measures make these preliminary findings all the more striking. Further, although the sample was selected randomly, and care was taken to convey an interest in the whole range of environmental attitudes, it is likely that some of those who elected not to participate were those who did not consider environmental issues to be of particular importance. Their scores on the ECS therefore may have been at the lower end of our sample. If the correlation found in this study is an accurate representation of a relationship, one would expect that some of these less environmentally oriented non-participants would have had low health scores as well. If that was the case, it is conceivable that our sampling could have contributed to a conservative correlation number.

What might the findings mean? The correlational nature of the study leaves as an open question the explanation of the relationship. For example, does personal health concern extend out to environmental concern? Does environmental concern lead to improved personal health behaviors, perhaps because of a greater perceived sense of control and potential for efficacy in the personal realm? Or are both attitudes and behaviors caused by a third variable, such as caring about the self or valuing life? Related, a third variable could be emotional health, reflected in part by a minimal need for denial. In any case, these results suggest that further exploration of the correlation found here could be informative to both areas of study. If further investigation shows that positive health and environmental behaviors may be effectively promoted in similar ways, there is potential for each field to inform the other's behavior change research efforts.

Limitations of the Study

The generalizability of the results of this study is limited by the use of a small, homogeneous sample of women. As indicated above, the correlational design limits conclusions that can be drawn. Self-report measures provide limited accuracy. Social desirability bias typically skews self-report on health behaviors, and was likely to do so on the environmental measure as well. Although the described procedures hopefully minimized the degree to which participants would limit their reporting to strongly positive environmental attitudes, the choice of the study and the nature of the content must have made evident the researchers caring about the environment.

The Health Questionnaire was designed to be a rough indicator of health behaviors for this preliminary study. Although it has face validity, its reliability coefficient is low, and empirical validity has not been established. The HQ could have been more informative if gynecological and medical examinations were inquired about separately. Medical examinations do not always involve cervical examinations for early detection of cancer, while gynecological examinations typically do. Further, the range of healthful alcohol consumption use is not clearly or consistently established by the scientific community or clearly or consistently understood by the general public. Choices offered and scoring of alcohol consumption may not well represent the actual or perceived healthful to not healthful range of consumption. The changes made to the Environmental Concern Scale may have impacted its previously established empirical validity in unknown ways. It is also possible that updates that were *not* made resulted in reduced validity. For example, the term "wise use," which was left in the questionnaire as a pro-environmental phrase, has over the years come to be associated with an anti-environmental movement.

Finally, although the Environmental Concern Scale makes minimal inquiry regarding a few possible self-reported behaviors, it is primarily a measure of attitudes. Attitudes have been shown to have only a weak relationship to behaviors due to the many potential obstacles to action (Stern, 2000). Care should be used in extrapolating the findings to behaviors. While attitudes play a role in behavior, it should not be assumed that these women would act in real situations in the ways they reported that they would act, or in ways one might think women with particular attitudes would act. Addressing each of these shortcomings will be important for future investigations.

Implications for Future Research

The significant relationship between health behaviors and environmental concern found in this preliminary study suggest that additional research needs to be conducted to confirm and then further our understanding of this relationship. A study utilizing a large and representative sample would allow analysis of various dimensions of the relationship, including possible variations on demographic variables such as age and race. Since attitudes are only partially predictive of behaviors, future studies may be most fruitful by looking at the relationship between health behaviors and actual environmental behaviors. Additionally, to the extent possible, it would be preferable to measure actual, as opposed to self-report, behaviors.

One potentially interesting future study might look at mammography and environmental behaviors. Most of the women in the current sample who had not had their examinations or mammograms within the year expressed awareness that they were late in doing so. They did not take action despite awareness of the need. A woman in a pilot investigation not only declined to pursue preventative testing, but she even avoided speaking with a doctor when experiencing likely symptoms of cancer. Women's avoidance of actions needed to verify the diagnosis and, if needed, to pursue treatment, may correspond to people's avoidance of actions to verify the extent of, and then to treat, environmental problems. For example, this woman's explanation that she did not like the treatment options so would rather do nothing certainly sounds similar to common industrial or political statements about various environmental protections or treatments not being economically feasible. In each case, if the problem is acknowledged, undesired treatment ought to follow; the problem is therefore ignored.

Similarly, this woman did receive occasional exposure from friends or newspapers to information that would encourage treatment, but explained it away or otherwise ignored it. Shaw (1982) wrote that when people are stressed with new information that leads to dissonance, they might simply keep themselves from thinking about it. Roszak (1993) wrote about the environmental condition as possibly being too overwhelming and frightening to face, so feelings and consequently further information gathering and action get shut down. Rothman et al. (1993) studied women over 40 who had not had mammograms during the prior year and found that those who did report feeling sad or scared in response to their encouraging educational presentation, as well as those with a sense of internal responsibility, were more likely to follow up with mammograms.

The woman's other explanation for her inaction was that she lacked faith in doctors. She did not take action because she did not believe her efforts would be effective. Similarly, Greenwald (1992) quotes a participant talking about pollution: "I feel like there isn't a lot I can do to change it. So it's something that I don't think about. It's one of those things that you kind of put off over there, that I can't do anything about it, so I won't think about it." Stern (2000) and others (McKenzie-Mohr, 2000; Winter, 2000) report that while information and consistent values/attitudes play some role in positive environmental actions, the more essential variables are ease of action (including no difficult barriers to overcome), and positive contingencies. Perceived consequences of action for the two women were not stronger and or more positive than those perceived for inaction. When the woman with cancer finally did experience so much pain that she had to face it and attempt treatment, she knew that she had let the problem go so long that a cure might no longer be possible. This certainly has parallels with the common denial of environmental problems until their impact has become visible (medical waste washes ashore), problematic (flooding occurs where wetlands were destroyed), costly, and possibly irreversible.

An additional question is whether fear of death may contribute to the denial. Many people will not buy coffins or even life insurance, perhaps saying, "I don't want to think about it." If we cannot face our own life cycle, the inevitability of our own death, it makes sense that it would be even more difficult to allow ourselves to think about the death of humanity or of Earth. Does it not make sense, then, that people would not want to think about or believe in global risks such as ozone depletion or global warming? It is commonly held in the social psychology literature that people underestimate their own vulnerability (Slovic, Fischoff, & Lichtenstein, 1982; Tversky & Kahneman, 1974). Perhaps this applies to people's estimation of their vulnerability in the context of environmental degradation as well. An in-depth study looking at women's feelings, attitudes, and behaviors with selected environmental issues and mammography could be informative with regard to many of these factors.

In summary, many challenges to behavioral change are similar, whether considering behaviors directly related to one's health and/or behaviors related to the health of the environment. Reasons underlying the challenge seem similar as well. In each case, factors limiting positive action may in part relate to denial, despair, feelings of invulnerability, awareness of barriers to effectiveness, external attribution for change, and a perception of the consequences of inaction as being more palatable than the consequences of action. Correlates of pro-health/environmental behaviors may include caring for the self, a more realistic appraisal of vulnerability, information seeking, and a sense of personal responsibility, self-efficacy, and hope. Further explorations of variables that are found to impact one or the other of environmental or physical health behaviors may warrant study in relation to the other.

Finally, an interesting question for future exploration would be whether interventions that successfully result in increased awareness and action in caring for the self would have a ripple effect resulting in increased action and caring for the environment, and, similarly, if environmental behavior change would lead to personal health behavior change.

Implications for Social Work

The findings of this study suggest that there is a link between personal health behaviors and environmental concern. This connection across what could seem to be two separate systems offers support for social work's ecological perspective with its person-in-environment approach. When using the person-in-environment approach, social work has tended to focus on the social and built world aspects of the person/environment exchanges. It appears that addressing the importance of the natural world/person exchange as well could improve the health both of the individual and of the environment. Park (1996) provides a useful example in her suggestion that social workers could use the earth interactively as a therapeutic tool. She writes that engaging clients in wilderness and other outdoor programs helps them to see the non-linear relationship between people and their world, thus developing a new way of knowing that respects and heals both the self and the environment. Social work interventions that are directly aimed at increasing people's positive health related behaviors may, in fact, have a "ripple effect" that increases the likelihood that people will, in turn, take action in their larger environments. Whether this is because of a direct connection between the environmental and health domains, or because of a third variable related to both, it may be useful for social workers helping people improve their personal health behaviors also to help them to see how the relevant skills and efforts can be transferred to other areas of concern.

For many years, social work has played an important role raising public awareness that understanding and helping individuals requires consideration of the wider context in which the individual lives, with which the individual interacts, and upon which the individual depends. This wider context as has typically been addressed has included familial, cultural, societal, and physical environment. Perhaps it is time for that understanding to be further broadened to include the importance of the relationship between the individual and the ecological environment. The centrality of the person-in-environment focus of social work practice puts social work in a natural position for addressing this connection as well as for bringing to the public an understanding of its relevance. Given the urgency of the global environmental condition, it may be important for social work to participate in addressing this relationship.

REFERENCES

Cohen, D., Scribner, R., & Farley, T. (2000). A structural model of health behavior: A pragmatic approach to explain and influence health behaviors at the population level. *Preventive Medicine: An International Journal Devoted to Practice & Theory, 30*(2), 146-154.

Dunlap, R., & Van Liere, K. (1984). Commitment to the dominant social paradigm and concern for environmental quality. *Social Science Quarterly, 65,* 1013-1028.

Gardner, G. T., & Stern, P. C. (1996). Environmental problems and human behavior. Needham Heights, MA: Allyn & Bacon.

Germain, C. B., & Gitterman, A. (1996). *The life model of social work practice: Advances in theory & practice* (2nd ed.). New York: Columbia University Press.

Greenwald, J. (1992). Environmental attitudes: A structural developmental model (Doctoral dissertation, University of Massachusetts at Amherst, 1992). *Dissertation Abstracts International, 53,* 6550B. (University Microfilms No. 82-06, 181).

Howard, G. (2000). Adapting human lifestyles for the 21st century. *American Psychologist, 55*(5), 509-515.

Janz, N. K., & Becker, M. H. (1984). The health belief model: A decade later. *Health Education Quarterly, 11*(1), 1-47.

Linsday, J., & Strathman, A. (1997). Predictors of recycling behavior: An application of a modified health belief model. *Journal of Applied Social Psychology, 27*(20), 1799-1823.

McKenzie-Mohr, D. (2000). Fostering sustainable behavior through community-based social marketing. *American Psychologist, 55*(5), 531-537.

Miller, S., Shoda, Y., & Hurley, K. (1996). Applying cognitive-social theory to health-protective behavior: Breast self-examination in cancer screening. *Psychological Bulletin, 119*(1), 70-94.

Oskamp, S. (2000). A sustainable future for humanity? How can psychology help? *American Psychologist, 55*(5), 496-508.

Park, K. (1996). The personal is ecological: Environmentalism of social work. *Social Work, 41*(3), 320-323.

Robbins, J., & Greenwald, R. (1994). Environmental attitudes conceptualized through developmental theory: A qualitative analysis. *Journal of Social Issues, 50*(3), 29-47.

Roszak, T. (1993). *The voice of the earth.* New York: Simon & Schuster.

Rothman, J., Salovey, P., Turvey, C., & Fishkin, S. (1993). Attributions of Responsibility and Persuasion Increasing Mammography Utilization Among Women Over 40 with an Internally Oriented Message. *Health Psychology, 12*(1), 39-47.

Shaw, M. (1982). *Theories of Social Psychology.* NY: McGraw-Hill.

Slovic, P., Fischoff, B., & Lichtenstein, E. (1982). Facts versus fears: Understanding perceived risk. In D. Kahneman, P. Slovic, & A. Tversky (Eds.), *Judgement under uncertainty: Heuristics and biases.* Cambridge, England: Cambridge University Press.

State of the world 1999-millennial edition: A world-watch institute report on progress toward a sustainable society. Brown, L., Flavin, C., French, H., Abramovitz, J., Dunn, S., Gardner, G., Mattoon, A., Platt McGinn, A., O'Meara, M., Renner, M.,

Roodman, D., Sampat, P., Tuxill, J., & Starke, L. (Eds.) (1999). Washington, D.C.: Worldwatch Institute.

Stern, P. (2000). Psychology and the science of human-environment interactions. *American Psychologist, 55*(5), 523-530.

Stern, P., Young, O., & Drickman, D. (Eds.). (1992). *Global environmental change: Understanding the human dimensions.* Washington, DC: National Academy Press.

Tversky, A., & Kahneman, D. (1974). Judgement under uncertainty: Heuristics and biases. *Science, 185,* 1124-1131.

Walker, J. M. (1979). Energy demand behavior in a master-meter apartment complex: An experimental analysis. *Journal of Applied Psychology, 64,* 190-196.

Weigel, R., & Weigel, J. (1978). Environmental concern: The development of a measure. *Environment and Behavior, 10,* 3-15.

Wilson, M., Daly, M., Gordon S., & Pratt, A. (1996). Sex differences in valuations of the environment? *Population & Environment: A Journal of Interdisciplinary Studies, 18*(2), 143-159.

Winter, D. (2000). Some big ideas for some big problems. *American Psychologist, 55*(5), 516-522.

APPENDIX
Health Questionnaire

For each of the following questions, circle the appropriate response:

1. During the past month, on average, how many days <u>per week</u> did you have one or more drinks of wine, beer, or other liquor?

   0   1-2   3-4   5-7

2. In the past month, on average, on the days when you drank alcoholic beverages, how many drinks did you have <u>per day</u>?

   1   2   3-4   5 or more   NA

3. On average, how many cigarettes do you smoke in a day?

   0   1-10   11-20   21 or more

4. During the past month, on average, how many days <u>per week</u> did you exercise for at least 20 minutes?

   0   1-2   3-4   5 or more

5. When in a car during the last week, how often did you wear your seat belt?

   Never   Once in a while   Most of the time   Every time

What is the approximate date (month and year) of your most recent physical or gynecological examination (i.e., your last check-up at the doctor's)?

_____

What is the approximate date of your most recent mammogram (breast x-ray)? If you have never had one, write "NA" for "not applicable"_____

APPENDIX (continued)

Health Questionnaire: Scoring System

Drinks/Week (= days drinking/week × drinks/day)

Category:	0	1-4	5-8	9 or more
Score:	4	3	2	1

Cigarettes/Day

Category:	0	--	1-10	11 or more
Score:	4	--	2	1

20 Minutes Exercise/Week

Category:	3 or more	1-2	0	--
Score:	4	3	2	--

Frequency Seatbelt

Category:	Every Time	Most of the Time	Once in a While	Never
Score:	4	3	2	1

Most Recent Gynecological Exam and Most Recent Mammogram (each scored as follows, and then the two scores are averaged for final score)

Category:	12 Mos. or Less	> 12 Mos. < 18 Mos.	> 18 Mos. < 24 Mos.	24 Mos. or More or Never
Score:	4	3	2	1

American Indian Women
and Domestic Violence:
The Lived Experience

Sharon B. Murphy
Christina Risley-Curtiss
Karen Gerdes

SUMMARY. During the past 25 years we have witnessed the growth and establishment of domestic violence as a field of inquiry. What has been noticeably absent, however, is research that explores the experience of American Indian women survivors of domestic violence. The data for this study were gathered from audiotaped, in-depth phemonenological interviews with 13 women from 10 American Indian Nations. This paper reports the findings of the study with particular emphasis on the uncovering of a spiral as a visual representation of the ways in which a woman is both entrapped by, and escapes from, domestic violence. Additionally, implications for social work practice with American Indian women, policy, and research are presented.

Sharon B. Murphy, PhD, is Domestic Violence Consultant, Arizona State University Faculty Associate, School of Social Work, Tempe, AZ 85287-1802.

Christina Risley-Curtiss, PhD, is Associate Professor, and Karen Gerdes, PhD, is Associate Professor, Arizona State University, School of Social Work, Tempe, AZ 85287-1802.

[Haworth co-indexing entry note]: "American Indian Women and Domestic Violence: The Lived Experience." Murphy, Sharon B., Christina Risley-Curtiss, and Karen Gerdes. Co-published simultaneously in *Journal of Human Behavior in the Social Environment* (The Haworth Social Work Practice Press, an imprint of The Haworth Press, Inc.) Vol. 7, No. 3/4, 2003, pp. 159-181; and: *Women and Girls in the Social Environment: Behavioral Perspectives* (ed: Nancy J. Smyth) The Haworth Social Work Practice Press, an imprint of The Haworth Press, Inc., 2003, pp. 159-181. Single or multiple copies of this article are available for a fee from The Haworth Document Delivery Service [1-800-HAWORTH, 9:00 a.m. - 5:00 p.m. (EST). E-mail address: docdelivery@haworthpress.com].

Digital Oject Identifier: 10.1300/J137v7n03_10

KEYWORDS. American Indian, domestic violence, phenomenology

Yearly estimates of the incidence of domestic violence in the United States vary widely but have not changed since the early studies were conducted during the 1970s and 1980s. Those estimates range from 1,000,000 (McCue, 1995) to 6,000,000 (Straus & Gelles, 1986) to the American Medical Association's estimate of 8,000,000-12,000,000 (Flitcraft, Hadley, Hendricks-Matthews, McLeer, & Warshaw, 1992). For the purposes of this study, violence against women and domestic violence are used interchangeably.

Although discrepancies exist regarding incidence rates of violence against women, researchers, academicians, and practitioners working in the field of domestic violence agree on several areas: (a) violence against women includes not only physical abuse but sexual, financial, psychological, and emotional abuse as well (Bograd, 1988; Pagelow, 1984; Pence & Paymar, 1993; Schechter, 1982; Walker, 1979, 1984); (b) domestic violence increases in both frequency and severity over time (Dobash & Dobash, 1984; Gelles, 1976; Pahl, 1985); and (c) the phenomenon of domestic violence has existed for a very long time and is a significant social problem within the United States today (Burge, 1989; Flitcraft, Hadley, Hendricks-Matthews, McLeer, & Warshaw, 1992; Glazer, 1993; U. S. Senate Judiciary Committee, 1992).

American Indian families have not been immune to this violence. Several studies have documented the existence of domestic violence as a social problem among American Indian people living both on and off reservations (Allen, 1985; Chapin, 1990; McIntire, 1988; Poelzer & Poelzer, 1986; Wolk, 1982). Each of the studies place the social problem of domestic violence in Indian Country within an historical framework. None of the studies to date, however, have attempted to examine the meaning of domestic violence from the perspective of the victims. The purpose of this paper is to provide a brief overview of the incidence of domestic violence in American Indian families, to report on a study of the lived experience of domestic violence among a sample of American Indian women, and to discuss implications of the study findings for policy, practice, and research.

DOMESTIC VIOLENCE AMONG AMERICAN INDIAN WOMEN

There is limited research on domestic violence within American Indian families. Much of the information that has been collected focuses on determining the scope of the problem. This appears to follow the path of early domestic violence research on the general United States population conducted between the mid 1970s through the 1980s (Straus, 1979; Straus & Gelles, 1986, 1990; Straus, Gelles, & Steinmetz, 1976, 1980). Additionally, research on domestic violence within the lives of American Indians often relies predominantly on quantitative methodologies, sometimes using assessment scales not designed for multicultural application (Chester, Robin, Koss, Lopez, & Goldman, 1994).

One of the inherent difficulties in collecting data on the size and scope of the problem within American Indian communities is that each American Indian tribe is a sovereign nation and as such collects data for its own purposes–not necessarily in the same manner across Indian country. Currently there are approximately 550 federally recognized tribes (Greenfield & Smith, 1999) within the United States, each with its own unique culture, language and history. Large scale national surveys such as those conducted by the U.S. Department of Justice are not designed to calculate incidence rates for each tribe. Therefore, most research is limited to individual American Indian nations and may not be generalizable to other Indian nations (Hamby & Supien, 1998).

Despite these difficulties, attempts have been made to quantify the problem of domestic violence among American Indians. The Minnesota Department of Corrections reported that American Indian women utilized battered women's shelters at 14 times their proportion of the state population (McIntire, 1988). The Minnesota study also found that domestic violence affected an estimated 50% of American Indian families (Wolk, 1982). Although Chapin's (1990) source of information is unclear, he reported that approximately 80% of the American Indian families in urban areas had a history of family violence. Bachman (1992) found 15.5% of American Indian couples reported violence in their relationship as compared to 14.8% of white couples. Zion and Zion (1993) reported that approximately 0.6 to 1% of Navajo adults are victims of domestic violence. Bohn (1993), and Norton and Manson

(1995) have conducted studies of domestic violence among American Indians seeking health care. Those studies revealed rates of domestic violence from 46% to 70%. Bohn also found, among a subgroup of 30 pregnant women, that 90% of the women had experienced some form of abuse.

In a study of abused children and their families at a southwestern area Indian Health Service hospital, researchers found that 76% of the adults reported domestic violence victimization (De Bruyn, Lujan, & May, 1992). Finally, a study conducted at a five-state American Indian regional psychiatric center found approximately 80% of the women treated at this facility had been victimized by sexual assault (Old Cross Dog, 1982). This report also noted the existence of sexual victimization among battered women.

A recent report by the U.S. Department of Justice (Greenfield & Smith, 1999) found that the rate of violent victimization among American Indians is more than double that of the general U.S. population (124 per 1,000 as compared to 50 per 1,000 persons age 12 or older). More than half of the violent victimizations of American Indians involved offenders with whom the victim had a prior relationship. Specifically, one in six violent victimizations involved an offender who was either an intimate or family member.

While still limited, our knowledge of the scope of domestic violence among American Indians is growing. However, our qualitative understanding of family violence within and among American Indian nations has only just begun. Domestic violence research within the majority society is approximately twenty-five years old. By contrast, the oldest identifiable study of domestic violence among American Indian couples is approximately sixteen years old. The bulk of the American Indian research has been conducted within the past eight to ten years. No studies were located which sought to uncover the personal meaning of domestic violence among American Indian women.

CURRENT STUDY

The Heideggerian hermeneutic phenomenological approach (Diekelmann & Allen, 1989) was used to investigate the lived experience of American Indian women survivors of domestic violence. This philosophy and methodology is ultimately concerned with the meanings that individuals make of their experiences, always acknowledging that meanings are embedded within a particular historical and cultural context. Phenomenology focuses on meanings through description and interpretation; it does not look for statistical relationships among variables nor frequencies of certain events or behaviors. It incorporates context and historicity which feminists (Dobash & Dobash, 1979) have long sought to include in studies of battered women. The goal of this form of inquiry is to understand the practical, everyday, common shared experiences.

METHODOLOGY

Study Setting

The study site was a residential substance abuse treatment facility for women and their children in a large southwestern metropolitan area. The goal of this center is to provide holistic treatment, including substance abuse treatment and domestic violence services, to American Indian women and their children. The facility serves a 40-tribe-wide area designated by the U.S. Indian Health Service. The study was a collaborative effort between the agency personnel and the primary author, who was serving as a domestic violence consultant to the agency at the time of the study.

Sample

The counseling staff at the treatment center described the study to those clients who had a history of domestic violence. The names of those clients who expressed an interest in participating were then given to the researcher to contact for assessment interviews to determine appropriateness and consent for the study. Counselors chose the date and times of the interviews so as not to interfere with the women's prescribed treatment program. Thirteen women volunteered to participate in the study. Each of the women received $25.00 compensation for participating in the study. The researcher was the recipient of a scholarship from the Ft. McDowell Mohave/Apache Indian Community which was used, in part, to reimburse the participants.

Each participant received written and oral information regarding the process of the interview, and the purpose of the research. Each woman was asked to complete the Participant Information Form and was asked to record a fictitious name by which she would be known throughout the study. Additionally, each woman was given an informed consent form and confidentiality statement, which was signed prior to the interview.

The following safeguards were established to diminish any uncomfortable feelings the women might experience after the interviews were completed: (a) night staff were given an interview schedule each day so that they could be available for any additional support; (b) the clinical supervisor or counseling staff members were on-call 24 hours a day for additional support; and (c) the researcher spent an additional hour following the interview processing any feelings regarding the interview or any content issues with each participant.

Data Collection

Interviews were conducted by the primary author at the treatment facility from May to September, 1997. The phenomenological interview was selected as a means of bringing the experience of domestic violence to the forefront. The guiding research question was: What is the lived experience of domestic violence of American Indian women survivors? The initial interview questions were: (a) What does the term domestic violence mean to you? and (b) Tell me a story about your domestic violence experience, one you will never forget. Each interview lasted approximately two hours or until the participant felt that she had told her story. Each interview was audiotaped and transcribed into a written text by the researcher.

Analysis

The method of investigation was analysis of in-depth phenomenological interviews. The computer software MARTIN (Diekelmann, Schuster, & Lam, 1994) was used to record the emerging themes. MARTIN is a data organizing tool for qualitative analysis, designed specifically to be used with hermeneutic studies. Heideggerian hermeneutics is both a philosophy and a methodology for extending human understanding by disclosing issues of meaning and subjective perception (Benner, 1994). The uniqueness of this methodology is its inclusion of others, i.e., research team and other members of the broader community, into the course of interpretation. This inclusionary process accepts the philosophical position that there are multiple meanings and that the uncovering of meanings combines many voices alongside the voice of the individual participant.

During the early stages of the analytic process, a research team was brought together to read the transcripts of the women's stories and to uncover emerging themes. Members of the research team included a nurse administrator and two American Indian social workers. Throughout the process of gathering emerging themes from the interview transcripts, the team constantly sought to ensure that the themes were warranted by the texts (transcripts). For example, each of the meetings with the research team (as well as research memos) was audiotaped and transcribed by the researcher. Transcriptions of interview texts, research team meetings, and research memos formed the corpus data of approximately 150 pages.

As the analytic process unfolded, the primary author wrote interpretations of the stories. These were given to several of the participants, several domestic violence experts, members of the American Indian community (both professionals in domestic violence and in other fields), several formerly battered women who were not participants in the study, and several experts in Heideggerian hermeneutic research. Input was sought from those readers for verification of completeness, coherence, comprehensiveness, and thoroughness of interpretations.

FINDINGS

Demographics

The study sample consisted of 13 American Indian women, each with a history of domestic violence and substance abuse. They came from ten American Indian nations (Colorado River Indian Tribes, Hopi, Morongo, Navajo, Paiute, Salt River Pima-Maricopa Indian Community, San Carlos Apache, Tohono O'Odham, White Mountain Apache, and Zia Pueblo) and ranged in age ranged from 23 to 48 years. Their levels of education ranged from completion of the 8th grade to two years of college. All but one woman had children, and the number of children in the family ranged from 1 to 7. Eight of the women were raised on reservations and 4 of those 8 women were raised speaking their tribal language. None of the women who were raised in urban settings spoke their native language as a first language. Eight of the 13 women were living on reservation land at the time of the study: Three of them described the setting as remote, as opposed to living within a community.

Six of the women stated that they practiced "traditional ways" prior to entering treatment at this facility. "Traditional ways" referred to participating in sweat lodge, and attending the Native American Church. Other spiritual beliefs practiced by the participants included membership in various Christian Churches (n = 5). Two of the women stated that they did not practice any religion.

Almost all (n = 12) of the women in this study had been in counseling prior to entering this treatment facility. Eight of the 12 women who had received prior counseling had been treated for substance abuse. Other issues that had been the focus of treatment in prior settings included general mental health problems (n = 7), child sexual abuse issues (n = 5), and depression (n = 5). One participant stated she had received counseling services while in a detention center for gang-related activities during adolescence. Of the 12 women who had received counseling services prior to entrance into the current treatment program, all had been victims of domestic violence, yet only one woman reported that a counselor asked about the presence of domestic violence in her relationship.

The common threads found among this diverse group of women were that each of them had experienced severe trauma, all were in recovery from drug and alcohol addiction, and all had survived domestic violence.

Content of the Stories

Each of the women in this study told stories of extraordinary physical and emotional abuse: All the stories were painful to speak and difficult to hear. During the time in which the violence took place, all of the women feared for their lives on a daily basis. All of the women vividly described being isolated, confused, feeling crazy, suicidal, fearful, and being trapped.

Constitutive Pattern

The themes "Breaking Down," "Breaking Out," and "Breaking Through" were uncovered in this study. Together, they suggest a constitutive pattern which we will call Claiming their Lives: A Spiral Journey of Survival. "Claiming" refers to the ways each woman in the study had taken over, taken charge of, and asserted ownership of her own life. The images that emerge from the women's stories contain both repetition and change, entrapment and hope. All of the women experienced repeated abusive acts by their partners but with each experience, the survivor managed to move–if only slightly–toward freedom. One way to conceptualize the pathway is through the image of a spiral: by tracing the circular path of her confinement, each woman moved up and down inside the spiral ultimately moving to the top. Protruding from the top of the spiral is a tall, thin spire. Some of the women can be seen teetering back and forth while balancing precariously on the top of the spire.

Helen states: " . . . what if he gets out [jail] tomorrow or something. I always ask myself that question, if he gets out I wonder if I'll go back with him." Others, such as Candace, the paradigm case in this study, can be seen using the spire as a springboard to freedom. The themes that have emerged in this study bring to light the experience of abuse and uncover the spiral as a common shared experience of the women participants.

Themes

The first theme, Breaking Down, describes the women's experience of victimization. In each case during breakdown the women can be seen winding their way up and down inside a spiral. Often, the women appear trapped by fear of impending danger and by a loss of self. "Losing self" has been described by the participants as having both internal and external manifestations. The internal or "feeling" manifestations of losing self include: confusion, abandonment, shame, suicidality, craziness, isolation, loss of reality and security, depression, and feeling trapped. External manifestations include circling and entrapment. Circling has been uncovered as a pattern of movement by the victim around her partner and around the bottom of the spiral. The practices of circling that have been identified are: maintaining physical closeness to her partner, hiding from him, standing guard over feelings, and moving around the partner's moods and violent outbursts. This theme reveals the absence of perception of choice and freedom as a component of the abusive relationship.

For Sarai, breakdown means being trapped, being alone, and total loss of spirit:

> . . . I was afraid to leave because I wouldn't have nobody. I'd be alone, he'd take my children which he did. It even got to the point where I prayed all the time . . . I prayed that my marriage would work . . . so I sat and waited for the day that my marriage would get better. Where it got to the point where I was nothing, I gave him my soul . . . my spirit . . . and I was nothing . . . I had nothing . . .

In the following excerpt Betty describes loss of self as confusion beginning in childhood:

> I've seen them [family members], just a lot of disturbance and I just stayed with my grandpa and grandma and after the next day things didn't look like it happened and they'd be all together again

and I started getting confused. At one time they were mad at each other, fighting, and the next day everything was nice and quiet where it seemed like nothing happened.

For Jean, loss of self reveals itself in suicidal thoughts:

> I think a part of me wanted to die but I was too scared to do it myself . . . I think that has a lot to do with the domestic violence too. Just looking for somebody to do what I can't do for myself.

External manifestations of losing self include the practice of circling. At the bottom of the spiral the women may be seen circling their spouses as they try to understand and react to his moods and violent outbursts. The women are constantly seeking ways to accommodate their partners as they search for safe places for self. For Candace, circling involved reading her partner's moods and looking for ways to be safe:

> If I stay with him, right next to him, he knows where I am and he can't accuse me of doing nothing behind his back, so it's safer to be with him sometimes even though you know you're gonna be beaten. It's not as bad as if he accuses you and beats you worse.

Candace also described how remaining physically close to her abusive partner helped her to maintain a modicum of safety. As Candace relayed this part of the story she showed me how she would stand physically close to her partner when she was particularly frightened that he would beat her. Candace explained that if she stood very close to him it became physically more difficult for him to reach her with his fist. She also believed that by standing near him she could distract him by showing him that she wanted to be close to him, thereby dissuading him from hitting her.

The second theme, Breaking Out, uncovered how the women in this study climbed up and out of the spiral and found themselves again. This theme represents the many ways the women moved beyond victimization to claim self. Included in this theme were the ways the women in this study climbed up the spiral through the shared practices of seeking distance from the relationship, crossing over from victim to survivor, and fighting back.

Some of the women, such as Ashley, noted that there was a particular point in time in which they became aware that they were victims. Ashley reported that during her pregnancy and later abortion, she noticed that the relationship had changed. Ashley's story continued with a description of how the process of crossing over from victim to survivor became stretched out over several months:

> And I started trying to leave him when he was sleeping or something. . . . First time I took a hundred dollars and went to stay in a motel and stayed there until he found me . . . From March to July I was running away from him and he was always coming back to get me. And then in June I . . . ran into an old friend from college and she didn't recognize me when she first saw me . . . I couldn't talk to her I just cried . . . She gave me her phone number and told me to call . . . and one night he came home and for no reason, I was laying in bed, he came in and he pulled me out of bed and started hitting me and kicking me and I didn't do anything. And he sat on the bed and all he said to me was, "Why are you still here?!" And he laid down and went to sleep and I . . . left.

This theme also uncovered the ways in which the women participants found themselves through the practices of prayer, sweat lodge, and by returning to traditional ways. Coyote and Betty talked about their rediscovery of a spiritual life as intrinsic to their ability to move up and out of the spiral. Religious practices taught to them as children, but forgotten during the years of abuse and alcoholism, have been reclaimed as part of the process of breaking out.

Coyote described a very painful childhood filled with abuse by her mother. As she mused about this part of her story and looked back over that relationship and the sadness that still remains, she talked about her faith in the power of the spirits. She spoke of the unfinished business between herself and her mother but expressed a belief that one day she will see her mother again:

> I think it's cause even up to the day that she died she never had a kind word to say to me and yet out of all the daughters I was the one that was up there up to the very end taking care of her because a part of me realized then that this was my mother that gave birth to me, that put me on this earth, and I loved her. I did! And this is kind of like unfinished business. I haven't heard from her. I deal with the spirits a lot and I see and I hear things . . . and I have not yet had the opportunity to have her come to me in a vision and tell me . . . that she was proud of me.

Betty found that by rediscovering her traditional beliefs her spirituality returned to her. Betty described getting back in touch with traditions as her source of strength. She stated: "And I got back in touch with my traditional [beliefs] and I started experiencing my spirituality . . . And there I found myself again." Rediscovering spirituality seems to have led to uncovering and discovering the meaning of the abusive experiences for several of the women in this study. Coyote also spoke of the power of prayer during her childhood, a practice she has recently revisited:

> She [mother] kicked me out in the middle of the night. And we lived like 7 miles from town and I walked in the darkness and I remember, cause, see my dad used to teach me, "pray, pray, pray." He'd take me out in the morning with my brothers and pray. And so when she used to kick me out like that I used to walk down the dark, dark road and pray. And it was scary and I'd call my dad, and it was like a miracle. "I'm over here! Coyote, I'm over here!" And he heard me, my prayers were answered, there was my father standing right in front of me! And he'd pick me up in total darkness and hold me.

The third theme, Breaking Through, revealed the process of moving from victim to victor as each of the women reached up and out of the spiral and onto the spire. Each of the women engaged in a reflective process as they told their stories, thus opening up the possibility of moving into new ways of being. By revisiting their former relationships, participants created new meanings (or truths) which expanded their horizons, creating new spaces, new dreams, and new hopes. The telling of the events of their lives opened up new possibilities for transforming self. As they looked back, they looked ahead.

For each of the women it was important to tell the events of the abusive relationship, to tell their story from beginning to end without interruption and in their own time frame. Uana found her voice the day she discovered her partner's infidelity and faced the impending end of the relationship. She described the scene in which she was able to break the silence:

> . . . and then one day I started crying and I couldn't stop . . . I was up all night crying and I knew I needed some kind of help . . . so I asked if she [mother] could give me a ride to the hospital . . . and the doctor . . . asked me if I thought it could wait until Monday [it

was Saturday] and that was one of the first times I ever spoke up for myself and I said that I couldn't [wait].

Finding voice and telling the story led to a process of reflection and thought for the future. Telling and listening to self engaged each of the women in the act of reflection allowing them to dwell within the stories as they wove them from beginning to end. Constitutive of the reflective process is Heidegger's concept of what it means to dwell (1959/1966). Jean approaches what Heidegger describes as "building dwelling thinking" (1971/1975) as she lives through or re-lives the violence, she dwells within it through the re-telling of her story and finally begins the thinking through or sorting out process. Jean engaged in reflective thought as she told her story of child sexual molestation by her father.

> God, it seems like that was one of the ways he showed it [love]. It wasn't, but it seems to me that I had to transform that abuse into love, because I had to as a little girl; it was a way of survival . . . And I think just being able to put everything together [telling her story], it happened . . . So now I know why, I think I can fix it. Maybe not fix it, I'll be able to heal, that's what I'll be able to do. I've never been able to do that before. I'm on a real strong road now; I've got a foundation to this thing and that just happened.

A Paradigm Story of Claiming Their Lives

Candace's story was chosen as the paradigm story because it most clearly reflected the experiences of the participants in this study. Within this story can be found the three themes as well as the constitutive pattern. Candace's story is about abuse which began during childhood, alcoholism, and a ten-year relationship with a severely emotional and physically abusive partner. That relationship ended almost ten years ago, but her partner's return to her reservation several years ago reawakened the fear that Candace had lived with for so long. This paradigm case is a story about victimization (Breaking Down) in which Candace moves around inside the spiral, circling, moving up and down, until ultimately reaching the spire (Breaking Out) and the springboard for claiming her life (Breaking Through).

> . . . he was the first love I ever had, he treated me real good. He was real nice to me, real kind to me, he was older than me, like 7 years older . . . he never hit me and I was really in love with him. And I

went away to school and then he used to write to me and ask me what I was doing. And I didn't know then but he was like controlling me and he was in prison. And that time he was in prison for assault I think, but he was in prison before for murdering somebody. And I just, I don't know, I loved this man a lot. I was okay with whatever he did cause I was gonna stick beside him . . . And everything was fine and then he started drinking a lot and I didn't drink . . . and then he would tell me . . . go ahead and drink and then I'd start drinking and then he'd get mad and say, "How come you don't talk to my friends, are you too good for my friends? And so we'd argue, well I won't argue with him; I'll just listen to him. And then he'll slap me and I'd think that was okay. . . Finally it just went on and he was hitting me more and more you know. I'd always hide my bruises and stuff like that . . . And I felt like . . . I loved him too much, that I couldn't leave him. He used to beat me up so bad you couldn't even see my nose cause it was so bruised . . . Then he'd always come back, always had some way of getting me back. He'd tell his friends and they'll come after me or something . . . cause I was learning to be scared of him and I didn't want to say no. And I felt like this was part of love that if I loved him I was supposed to be with him, and I was supposed to do whatever he wanted.

The beginning of Candace's story reveals her faithfulness to a man who initially was kind to her. For Candace, faithfulness to a man who had shown her kindness was translated into sticking beside him no matter what he had done. As she tells her story, she looks back and states that her abusive partner began to exert control over her in the earliest days of the relationship. His ability to cover up his abuse tactics took many forms over the years. Candace talked about being controlled through letters while he was in prison and she was away at high school. Being away at high school in Candace's case refers to attending a Bureau of Indian Affairs boarding school. Boarding schools are education programs designed by the federal government for American Indian children. They were intended to educate the children in the ways of the majority culture away from their homes and families (Duran & Duran, 1995). The boarding school that Candace attended was several hundred miles away from Candace's home on the reservation. The classes she attended were taught in English, and the children were not allowed to speak their tribal language nor practice Indian ways. Candace's partner's abusive tactics first began through letters.

Shortly after she returned to the reservation her boyfriend introduced her to alcohol and soon began to pressure her into drinking with him.

Physical assaults, intimidation, isolation from family and friends, and intense fear all contributed to her partner's extensive network of control and domination.

> . . . he said he wanted to go see a couple of his friends. The guy who was his friend was my classmate, we knew each other. So we went to his friend's house and we're all in the front seat of his car and he [boyfriend] got out to go see his friend and I didn't move over and I just sat beside this guy and then he [boyfriend] came back to the car and he was real mad. I could tell by his face. He was saying, "Take us back home, take us back home!" . . . we got off and I knew he was gonna fight and I was real scared. And he goes, "How come you didn't move over, I seen you kissing him!" And I said, "No, I wasn't kissing him!" And then he goes, "Yeah, you were!" and then he hit me and he goes, "Bitch, I'm gonna take care of this once and for all!" He went inside the house and I walked right behind him . . . And I didn't know what to do . . . I knew if I went out then he'll beat me up and also I was just trying to be by him so that he won't . . . hurt me . . . and he picked up this knife . . . all I knew was that when I turned around I felt like something warm on my stomach . . . I didn't know what to do . . . I started walking off . . . I was gonna walk to the neighbors and have them call somebody cause I was 3 months pregnant. And I got to the butane tank and I couldn't walk no more.

As Candace stated earlier, " . . . he would tell me to go ahead and drink and then I'd start drinking and then he'd get mad and say, 'How come you don't talk to my friends, are you too good for my friends?' " For Candace, the introduction to alcohol and her partner's pressure to drink with him and his friends began the process of her addiction. Additionally, over time the abusive acts became increasingly severe and were coupled with a growing terror. As the abuse worsened she became increasingly isolated from family and friends. Candace's world shrank to her abusive partner, his friends, beatings, and alcohol. Breakdown is vividly portrayed in the following excerpt:

> And I said I don't want him anymore cause he beat me up too many times [and] I was aching to drink cause then that was the only thing that made me feel alright was when I drink cause it helped me forget. So we [Candace and her cousins] took off to the

store and then just when we got to the store, there was this car there and he was sitting in that car. And I got real scared and I said, "Turn around, let's go back, there he is!" And then they started chasing us and then that car pulled alongside us and this guy would say, "He [her abusive boyfriend] wants to talk to Candace!" And then I said, "No, no, no!" Then he pulled out that gun and he said "if you don't stop I'm gonna shoot you!" [and I knew] if I tried to leave him he would do something to me.

And later:

He would always say, "If I can't have you nobody can" and "Yeah, you think you're all pretty now, I'll scar up your face!" . . . he used to chase me all over and if I didn't go with him he'd fight somebody or whoever I was with so I was scared for my friends so I just have to go with him then he'll be nice to me . . . and I just didn't want to be with him and I told him, "This is it!" And I kept hiding out here and there. And then I went to a dance and he had hooked up with another girl and she started getting mad at me . . . And he said to his new girlfriend, "What are you doing, leave her alone!" And he stabbed that girl! . . . and that made me more and more scared of him cause he was there, he would go and come back and nobody could do nothing to him. There was no stopping him, if he wanted me then he was going to have me. I couldn't get away.

Isolated and living in complete terror, Candace felt that she had no recourse but to remain with him, fearing that if she tried to leave he would kill her. At this point of breakdown she states that she stopped caring for herself because she knew there was no way out for her. She remained in the relationship until the day her abusive partner was taken to jail on suspicion of murder. Candace took up a new residence away from the reservation, believing that creating distance would guarantee her safety. Soon, however, she discovered that the charges against her partner had been dropped, and he had been released from jail. She spent the next several years moving back and forth trying to find a safe place. She lived within the spiral, circling, looking for safety, moving up and down within the spiral. In a later interview, Candace discussed her breakdown: "You know, there's a spider spinning his web inside the spiral and sometimes you get stuck in its sticky stuff and sometimes it takes a long time to get loose from it."

Reclaiming self (Breaking Out) for Candace was a long slow process. She described many times that she had attempted to leave her partner by putting geographic distance between them, by hiding out on the reservation, by reporting his illegal activities to the police, and by assisting police through information that would aid in an arrest and conviction. It was during a period of several years in which Candace found safety from him that he reappeared.

It was at that time that she said:

> . . . I finally said, "No, no more!" and I wouldn't go back to him. I knew that I was worth something also. Before I was nothing; I was just his slave.

Candace talks about rediscovering her spirituality (Breaking Out) as a source of healing and as an integral component of reclaiming self (Breaking Through). Candace's spiritual life was reborn during her substance abuse treatment. In the following excerpt Candace talks about the power of telling her story (Breaking Through) intertwined with the power of her spiritual beliefs. She vividly describes moving out of the spiral and onto the spire:

> This morning at meditation I prayed that I would be okay doing this [telling her story] because I was afraid that when I told my story I might lose my mind . . . I thought if I re-lived it this time I might really lose my mind. So I asked for that strength . . . I knew my Creator would let me deal with it and not lose my mind.

For Candace, telling the story, remembering the events and re-living them, and listening to self led to the act of reflecting upon what had been:

> That sweat lodge has heard my story, those stones, the stone people, they're the ones who know everything about me. I prayed to them and I told them all the abuse I went through, they know and I prayed and I left it there and I never told another human being until today. So it doesn't have to be a secret anymore. Many times in sweat I purified, to take all the things I hid inside, the skeletons in my closet. That's why I asked the Creator today to give me the strength to tell my story and I prayed the four directions and I cried

cause I was scared. After I said my prayer I felt better, I knew that I'll be taken care of, the Creator never lets me down. And it's all over, and I'm still sitting here and I've still got my mind.

Her sense of spirituality became intimately connected with the reflective process. The act of reflection included dwelling within the story as Candace wove her story from beginning to end within her own time frame.

DISCUSSION AND IMPLICATIONS

The purpose of this study was to explore the lived experience of American Indian women victims of domestic violence. This study expands upon the existing body of literature by bringing to light the common experiences and shared practices among a group of American Indian women. The study adds to our understanding of the many ways in which women have been victimized, how they understand their victimization and live within it, and how they move out of it and into survivorhood.

Implications for Social Worker's Understanding of Human Behavior Knowledge

It is incumbent upon social workers to understand the worldview of the clients with whom we work. That worldview becomes clearer as we develop an awareness of our clients' culture, history, degree of traditionality, spirituality, and language. Understanding a client's worldview provides us with a context for understanding human behavior.

This study has revealed the spiral as a visual representation of the experience of the American Indian women in this study. The image is particularly helpful for non-Indian social workers working with American Indian battered women. Seeing life and human behavior from a circular dimension, a worldview that may be different from our own, adds depth to our understanding of a client's experience and another dimension to our own interpretive stance. The spiral offers social workers another interpretation for human behavior that removes the practitioner from the dualism of "either/or" thinking or what the client should or shouldn't do in terms of extricating oneself from a violent partner. Within the spiral are many twists and turns depicted graphically in the themes and paradigm case. The practices of circling were revealed as both loss of self but also as a means of protecting oneself from the violent partner. Within breakdown, the stories uncovered the various ways in which the women circled their partner, and were trapped. The practices associated with breakdown are just now becoming visible to the women as they weave their stories. Movement up and down the spiral and onto the spire is described in the second and third themes. Each theme contributes to our understanding of human behavior as defined by the context and environment in which the behavior occurs.

Social Work Practice Implications

There are a number of implications for social work practice that have evolved from the methodology of this study. Briefly, the interpretive phenomenological interview is non-directive, uses an open-ended invitation to each participant to tell her story, and is conversational in style. Consequently, use of this methodology meant allowing each woman to define her story and describe her experiences in terms of her own content, context, and use of language. That is, the interview itself empowered each woman. The interpretive phenomenological interview could be incorporated within the clinical interview to have a similar impact. Implications for practice based upon this methodology will be discussed in greater detail in a future article.

Other implications for social work practice have evolved directly from the women's stories. For example, each theme presents practitioners with new ways of thinking and responding to the needs of domestic violence victims and survivors. In addition, the results of this study supports the idea that in order to do "best practice," it is incumbent upon the social worker to understand the experience of being a victim as defined by the particular culture of the client. Practitioners' tasks include finding ways to facilitate breaking through and breaking out. Social workers can facilitate this movement by inviting their clients to tell their stories of breakdown. It is through these stories that clients' strengths are most visible. Each woman needs to be able to tell her story in her own way and in her own time. The matter of time deserves special focus for social workers assisting American Indian victims of domestic violence.

Time also refers to the length of time it may take an individual woman to come to the realization that she has been a victim of domestic violence. Social workers can assist women victims in determining when the time is right by conducting on-going assessments of levels of danger and degree of severity of abuse. That information needs to be shared with the client on a continuing basis. For those women who are afraid to leave because of the risk based upon the abusers' threats and past violence, it is critical that social workers provide supportive services, safety planning, and linkages with the criminal justice system.

Victims of domestic violence require varying lengths of time to reflect upon the abuse experience. Social workers need to allow each woman the time that she needs to move out of breakdown and into survival and healing. Acknowledging a woman's ability to know when it is right for her to leave plays an important role in empowering victims of domestic violence. The women in this study also talked about the ways in which they sought distance from the abuser, how they became aware of their victimization, and how they fought back. Practitioners can assist women victims by reframing the common practice of leaving and returning to the abusive relationship as a rehearsal for leaving for good, thereby reducing the clients' guilt or shame about having returned to her abusive partner. Each of the ways in which the women in this study sought distance from the abuse can be seen as signs of preparing to leave. Often women victimized by domestic violence seek answers for their behavior and confirmation of their experiences. Social workers armed with the knowledge of how the women in this study sought distance from the abuser and abusive relationship can assist other women victims.

The women in this study also talked about finding self through their traditional beliefs. Helping women to reconnect to cultural and traditional beliefs is another way of assisting the healing process. This may be especially important for those clients who have relocated to urban areas from predominantly rural communities. Helping clients to find those connections again, or to connect for the first time, can contribute to the healing process.

Implications for Social Work Policy

In relation to social policy, one of the major impediments to working effectively with American Indian women victims of domestic violence is the current climate of managed care. Often in managed care settings social workers are required to use assessment forms that limit or preclude open-ended questions. Additionally, assessment forms do not allow for a holistic approach to assessment. Rather, the specified questions focus attention on the purview of the specific agency. This means that other issues often go unidentified. Also, treatment practices dictated by managed care adhere to a highly structured (and often unrealistic) time frame. Non-pressured story telling as the primary means of healing, the treatment suggested by this research, does not fit within the paradigm of brief therapy.

Directions for Future Research

There is still much to be learned about domestic violence and American Indian women. Additional research needs to be done including replications of the current study. Studies that focus on the experiences of women who have been apart from the abusive relationship for a significant period of time may also give practitioners new information about the experience of domestic violence. Also, research on the experiences of women of color would add a new dimension to such studies. Future research might also evaluate the effects of cross-cultural training on social work practice within the context of domestic violence.

CONCLUSION

This study explored and described the experiences of thirteen American Indian women victims of domestic violence. It enhanced and expanded upon our understanding about victimization and survivorhood by bringing into light the common experiences and shared practices of women victims. The constitutive pattern expressed the relationship of each story to another and formed the over-arching pattern joining themes. The themes, Breaking Down, Breaking Out, and Breaking Through, uncovered the image of a spiral as the visual representation of victimization and survivorhood. The voices of the women participants in this study have brought to light a number of key areas to enhance social work practice as well as important issues to be raised in the arena of mental health policy.

REFERENCES

Allen, P. G. (1985). *Violence and the American Indian woman. The speaking profits us: Violence in the lives of women of color.* Seattle: Center for the Prevention of Sexual and Domestic Violence.

Annells, M. (1996). Hermeneutic phenomenology: Philosophical perspectives and current use in nursing research. *Journal of Advanced Nursing, 23*, 705-713.

Bachman, R. (1992). *Death and violence on the reservation.* NY: Auburn House.

Benner, P. (1994). The tradition and skill of interpretive phenomenology in studying in health, illness, and caring practices. In P. Benner (Ed.), *Interpretive phenomenol-*

ogy: Embodiment, caring, and ethics in health and illness. Thousand Oaks, CA: SAGE Publications.

Bograd, M. (1988). Feminist perspectives on wife abuse: An introduction. In M. Bograd & K. Yllo (Eds.), *Feminist perspectives on wife abuse* (pp. 11-26). Newbury Park, CA: SAGE Publications.

Bohn, D. (1993). Nursing care of Native American battered women. *AWHONN Clinical Issues, 4* (3), 424-434.

Burge, S. (1989). Violence against women as a health care issue. *Family Medicine, 21* (5), 368-373.

Chapin, D. (1990). Peace on earth begins in the home. *The Circle, 14,* 1.

Chester, B., Robin, R., Koss, M., Lopez, J., & Goldman, D. (1994). Grandmother dishonored: Violence against women by male partners in American Indian communities. *Violence and Victims, 9* (3), 249-258.

De Bruyn, L., Lujan, C., & May, P. (1992). A comparative study of abused and neglected American Indian children in the southwest. *Soc. Sci. Med., 35* (3), 305-315.

Diekelmann, N., & Allen, D. (1989). A hermeneutic analysis of the NLN criteria for the appraisal of baccalaureate programs. In N. Diekelmann, D. Allen, & C. Tanner, *The NLN Criteria for Appraisal of Baccalaureate Programs: A Critical Hermeneutic Analysis* (pp. 11-31). NY: National League for Nursing.

Dieklemann, N., Schuster, R., & Lam, S. (1994). MARTIN, a computer sofware program: On listening to what the text says. In P. Benner (Ed.), *Interpretive phenomenology: Embodiment, caring, and ethics in health and illness* (pp. 129-140). Thousand Oaks, CA: SAGE Publications.

Dobash, R. E., & Dobash, R. P. (1979). Violence against wives: A case against the patriarchy. In *Violence Against Wives* (pp. 1-13). NY: The Free Press.

Dobash. R., & Dobash, E. (1984). The nature and antecedents of violent events. *British Journal of Criminology, 24* (3), 269-288.

Duran, E., & Duran, B. (1995). *Native American postcolonial psychology.* Albany, NY: State University Press.

Flitcraft, A., Hadley, S., Hendricks-Matthews, M., McLeer, S., & Warshaw, C. (1992). American medical association diagnostic and treatment guidelines on domestic violence. *Archives of Family Medicine, 1,* 39-47.

Gelles, R. (1976). Abused wives: Why do they stay? *Journal of Marriage and the Family, 38* (4), 659-668.

Glazer, S. (1993). Violence against women. *CQ Researcher, 3,* 171.

Greenfield, L., & Smith, S. (1999). *American Indians and crime.* Washington, DC: U.S. Department of Justice, Bureau of Justice Statistics.

Hamby, S., & Supien, M. B. (1998). *Domestic violence on the San Carlos Apache Reservation: Rates, associated psychological symptoms, and current beliefs.* Paper presented at the 10th Annual HIS Research Conference, Albuquerque, NM.

Heidegger, M. (1966). Discourse on thinking. (J. M. Anderson & E. H. Freund, Trans.). NY: Harper & Row, Publishers. (Original work published 1959).

Heidegger, M. (1975). Poetry, language, thought. (A. Hofstadter, Trans.). NY: Harper & Row, Publishers. (Original work published 1971).

McCue, M. (1995). *Domestic violence a reference handbook.* Santa Barbara, CA: Contemporary World Issues.

McIntire, M. (1988). Societal barriers faced by American Indian battered women. *Women of Nations Newsletter*.

Norton, I., & Manson, S. (1995). A silent minority: Battered American Indian women. *Journal of Family Violence, 10* (3), 307-318.

Old Cross Dog, P. (1982). *Listening past*. Indian Health Service (April 1982).

Pagelow, M. (1984). *Family violence*. NY: Praeger Special Studies.

Pahl, J. (1985). *Private violence and public policy*. London: Routledge & Kegan Paul.

Palmer, R. (1969). *Hermeneutics*. Evanston, IL: Northwestern University Press.

Pence, E., & Paymar, M. (1993). *Education groups for men who batter*. NY: Springer Publishing Company.

Poelzer, D. T., & Poelzer, I. A. (1986). Women, marriage, and the family. In D. T. Poelzer & I. A. Poelzer, *In our own words: Northern Saskatchewan metis women speak out* (pp. 45-53). Saskatoon, Saskatchewan: Lindenblatt and Hamonic Publishing.

Schechter, S. (1982). *Women and male violence*. Boston: South End Press.

Straus, M. (1979). Measuring intrafamily conflict and violence: The Conflict Tactics (CT) Scales. *Journal of Marriage and the Family, 41*, 75-88.

Straus, M., & Gelles, R. (1986). Societal change and change in family violence from 1975 to 1985 as revealed by two national surveys. *Journal of Marriage and the Family, 48*, 465-479.

Straus, M., & Gelles, R. (Eds.). (1990). *Physical violence in American families: Risk factors and adaptation to violence in 8,145 families*. New Brunswick, NJ: Transaction Publications.

Straus, M., Gelles, R., & Steinmetz, S. (1976). *Violence in the family: An assessment of knowledge and research needs*. Paper presented at the American Association for the Advancement of Science, Boston, MA.

Straus, M., Gelles, R., & Steinmetz, S. (1980). *Behind closed doors*. Garden City, NY: Anchor Books.

United States Senate Judiciary Committee. (1992). *Violence against women*. Washington, D.C.: U.S. Government Printing Office.

Walker, L. (1979). *The battered woman*. NY: Harper Colophon Books.

Walker, L. (1984). *The battered woman syndrome*. NY: Springer Publishing Company.

Wolk, L. E. (1982). *Minnesota's American Indian battered women: The cycle of oppression; a cultural awareness training manual for non-Indian professionals*. St. Paul, MN: St. Paul Indian Center.

Zion, J. W., & Zion, E. B. (1993). Hozho "sokee"–stay together nicely: Domestic violence under Navajo common law. *Arizona State Law Journal, 25*, 407-426.

Women with Disabilities
and Experiences of Abuse

Elizabeth P. Cramer
Stephen F. Gilson
Elizabeth DePoy

SUMMARY. A qualitative study of disabled and non-disabled professionals and survivors of abuse revealed a range of types of abuse endured by disabled women, some of which were unique to that population. Two major themes emerged from data analysis: vulnerable beginnings and complexity of abuse. Three sub-themes are encompassed within complexity of abuse: active abuse, abuse through image, and contextual abuse by social service/legislative systems. The authors present data essential to an informed assessment and analysis of abuse that considers the person-in-environment circumstances of women with disabilities.

Elizabeth P. Cramer is Associate Professor, Virginia Commonwealth University.
Stephen F. Gilson is Associate Professor, University of Maine, Orono.
Elizabeth DePoy is Professor, University of Maine, Orono.
Address correspondence to: Dr. Elizabeth P. Cramer, Virginia Commonwealth University, P.O. Box 842027, 1001 West Franklin Street, Richmond, VA 23284-2027.

The authors would like to thank Elizabeth Hutchison for reviewing a draft of this article; Nancy Smyth for her insightful review of the article; Teresa Bsullak, Ellen Stevens, Raphael Mutepa, and Kris Hash for assisting with data collection and analysis; and the participants of the focus groups who shared generously of their personal and professional experiences.

[Haworth co-indexing entry note]: "Women with Disabilities and Experiences of Abuse." Cramer, Elizabeth P., Stephen F. Gilson, and Elizabeth DePoy. Co-published simultaneously in *Journal of Human Behavior in the Social Environment* (The Haworth Social Work Practice Press, an imprint of The Haworth Press, Inc.) Vol. 7, No. 3/4, 2003, pp. 183-199; and: *Women and Girls in the Social Environment: Behavioral Perspectives* (ed: Nancy J. Smyth) The Haworth Social Work Practice Press, an imprint of The Haworth Press, Inc., 2003, pp. 183-199. Single or multiple copies of this article are available for a fee from The Haworth Document Delivery Service [1-800-HAWORTH, 9:00 a.m. - 5:00 p.m. (EST). E-mail address: docdelivery@haworthpress.com].

10.1300/J137v7n03_11

Implications for future research and the human behavior in the social environment curriculum are discussed. *[Article copies available for a fee from The Haworth Document Delivery Service: 1-800-HAWORTH. E-mail address: <docdelivery@haworthpress.com> Website: <http://www.HaworthPress.com> © 2003 by The Haworth Press, Inc. All rights reserved.]*

KEYWORDS. Disability, abuse, domestic violence, women with disabilities, battering and disability

Although domestic violence has received a significant amount of attention in both the scholarly literature and the service sector, little targeted attention has been directed to abused women with disabilities in social work knowledge, curricula, and practice. Thus, there is a dearth of empirically-based theory and knowledge informing curriculum and practice with this neglected population of women. The research that has been done has suggested that a disproportionate number of disabled women[1] are subjected to abuse, and many women become disabled as a result of abuse. Building on recent work which revealed the important distinctions between abuse of disabled and nondisabled women, the study presented herein was designed to (a) explore and characterize abuse unique to women with disabilities, and (b) provide empirical knowledge on which to teach about, assess, develop, and provide services to abused women with disabilities.

The authors provide an overview of the literature on abused women with disabilities, describe the methodology used in the study, and present data essential to an informed assessment and analysis that considers the unique person-in-environment circumstances of women with disabilities. Second, the authors interpret the study's findings in light of the curriculum mandate to include knowledge about the experiences of marginalized and oppressed populations as populations at-risk for subjugation, denial of civil and legal rights, and both generalized and specific experiences of victimization. Lastly, the authors link the theory suggested herein to further theory development, research, and practice.

PREVALENCE OF ABUSE

In excess of three million women are physically abused by intimate partners each year, and nearly one-third (25-31%) of women in the U.S.

will have been physically or sexually abused by a husband or boyfriend at some point in their lives (Tjaden & Thoennes, 1998). The numbers of women abused increases when considering non-physical abuse, such as emotional abuse, threats of and actual intimidation, and controlling behaviors that regulate the actions, experiences, and circumstances of disabled women by the abuser. One subpopulation of domestic violence victims, women with disabilities, has received little attention in the domestic violence literature, although statistical examination reveals that they are at particular risk for physical and sexual abuse in their homes, in hospitals, and in institutions (Gilson, Cramer, & DePoy, in press; Nosek et al., n.d.; Sobsey, 1994).

While few prevalence studies on abused, disabled women have been conducted, there is some empirical research that illuminates the scope of the problem. It was revealed in a national study of 439 women with physical disabilities and 421 women who did not have disabilities that the rate of abuse experienced by disabled women and nondisabled women is comparable. The same percentage of both groups of women (62%) had experienced emotional, physical, or sexual abuse at some point in their lives. For both disabled and nondisabled women, husbands or live-in partners were the most common perpetrators of physical or emotional abuse. Compared to nondisabled women, women with disabilities experienced abuse for a longer duration, were more likely to be abused by a greater number of perpetrators, reported a higher number of health care workers and attendants as the perpetrators, and noted fewer options for escaping or resolving the abuse (Young, Nosek, Howland, Chanpong, & Rintala, 1997).

Consistent with the prevalence statistics, disabled women themselves have identified abuse as a serious personal concern. In a study of 100 disabled women, abuse and violence was ranked as their number one priority (Berkeley Planning Associates, 1992).

THE NEED FOR RESEARCH TO INFORM THEORY, CURRICULUM AND PRACTICE

The service and resource needs of abused, disabled women have just begun to be studied. However, due to the dearth of empirical knowledge about disability and abuse, there are major barriers to the development of theory and empirically based services and supports that can enhance inclusion, productivity, safety and quality of life for this population. Three particular areas have been noted as service barriers, due in large part to the absence of sound knowledge about the population: (a) incapacity to identify the unique abuse encountered by disabled women, (b) negative attitudes towards disabled women, and (c) inaccessibility of services.

Incapacity to Identify the Unique Abuse Encountered by Disabled Women

A primary barrier to addressing the needs of abused, disabled women is the recognition of the unique forms of abuse that they experience. Narrow definitions of physical abuse, such as a criminal justice definition of physical assault, may exclude those disabled women who are being abused by control and restraint, mechanisms that may appear to service providers to be less harmful in the nondisabled population than direct assault. Examples of these situations include withholding access to medications, controlling assistive devices, and refusing to communicate using assistive devices or with sign language (Gilson et al., in press).

Failure to recognize abuse may serve to isolate women from services and supports that could potentially decrease or eliminate the abuse and provide a supportive environment in which women with disabilities can live safely and productively. Furthermore, disabled women have noted that standard abuse assessments fail to identify the types and extent of abuse occurring in their relationships, and thus, providers using such instruments do not identify many abuse situations as domains for intervention (Gilson et al., in press).

Negative Attitudes

Women with disabilities note that they are sometimes disbelieved when they disclose the abuse to service providers, due, in part, to societal myths that perpetuate the view of women with disabilities as asexual, unlikely to be in a relationship, or unlikely to be abused because others would take pity on them rather than abuse them (Calvey, 1998). Chenoweth (1996), Gilson et al. (in press), and Sobsey (1994) note that when disabled women are taught to comply with the requests and instructions of others, they become silenced in expressing their true experiences and needs. Moreover, women in the Gilson et al. study reported difficulty communicating with service providers, including hotline staff, healthcare providers, and police, in large part due to dual service systems (disability services and domestic violence services) that separate "disability issues" and "domestic violence issues." For example, women reported contacting a domestic violence services agency, but once they identified themselves as having a disability they were immediately referred to the disability services agency in the community. The women reported that healthcare providers are trained to view disability, rather than abuse, as the issue for treatment.

Inaccessibility of Services

Domestic violence services (shelter and non-shelter) may be located in physically inaccessible settings, lack material available in alternative format, lack staff proficient in the use of American Sign Language, and lack the training to provide services on multiple cognitive receptive and expressive levels. Because para-transit services often operate on a limited schedule (daytime and weekdays) and ordinarily require advanced notice of request for transport, and shelter programs, generally, are unable to provide modified vehicles or other accessible transportation, women with disabilities who may require transportation support are seriously limited in their access to crisis and/or after hours safety and support services. Domestic violence programs may be unable to provide or coordinate personal care assistance for the woman needing such assistance to leave her home (National Coalition Against Domestic Violence, 1996).

The development of a knowledge and theory base that underpins informed person-in-environment teaching, assessment, and intervention will be key to thoughtful, effective, and responsive curriculum and practice for and with abused, disabled women. The study discussed below yields substantive data to anchor theory, curriculum, research, and practice.

METHODOLOGY

Literature about innovative, community-based methodology clearly highlights the limitations of traditional research paradigms for illuminating the nature of domestic violence and abuse for disabled women and distinguishing it from abuse common to all women (Gill, Kirschner, & Panko Reis, 1994; Gilson et al., in press). Consistent with ecological person-in-environment approaches, disability researchers have been calling for methodologies which are capable of revealing multi-perspective insights as a basis for theory and program development (Barnes & Mercer, 1997; Seelman & Sweeney, 1997).

Moreover, the population of abused, disabled women cannot be treated as homogeneous, since in addition to being varied in type and nature of disability, women with disabilities, like nondisabled women, hold membership in many communities and groups, such as those based on age, geographic location, ethnicity, sexual orientation, faith belief, and culture among others.

Because of the beginning stages of tested theory in this important topic of inquiry, naturalistic design relying on focus group interview and thematic and taxonomic data analysis was selected to build on previous inquiry for theory generation (DePoy & Gitlin, 1998). Focus group interviewing provides the context for group dynamics to generate reflection and stimulate thought allowing additional data to emerge that may not have emerged in individual interviews (Frey & Fontana, 1993) and allows for rich descriptions of process and meaning (Creswell, 1994).

The authors were also influenced by feminist interview research (Reinharz, 1992). Given that dominant groups have historically spoken for women, and people with disabilities, this methodology allows this population to tell and interpret their own experiences in their own words. Feminist interview research also encourages such feminist notions as establishing a rapport and relationship between interviewee(s) and interviewer, and use of personal self-disclosure, both of which were used in this study.

In sum, a fundamental premise of our research was that a group of women who experience abuse have not been studied extensively, cannot be characterized by theory developed from empirical information about nondisabled women, and thus require theory generation emerging from the uniqueness of this population (DePoy & Gitlin, 1998).

Data Collection and Analysis

Four focus group interviews were held in the spring of 1998 and winter and spring of 1999 in a state in the southeastern US: the first in an urban setting; the second in a small, rural town; the third in a small town in a mountain valley region; and the final group in a tobacco and textile town.

The following open-ended questions were posed to participants: (a) what forms of abuse occur most often among women with disabilities? (b) How can the woman with a disability(ies) protect herself and her children? (c) What could people and agencies in the community do to address the issue of abuse among women with disabilities and make reporting easier? (d) To conduct further research on abused women with disabilities, what could researchers do to gain access to the women, and what questions should researchers ask?

All four focus groups were organized by providing questions in writing and orally to participants. Because of the extensive discourse offered by participants, few probes to expand the discussion were necessary. Each group was audio taped, and tapes were subsequently transcribed verbatim. Field notes were also taken during each session. Specific accommodations to assure accessibility and full participation of individuals with hearing and/or sight impairments were used in all focus groups.

The researchers analyzed the focus group data through use of the computer program QSR NUD*IST (1996). The researchers engaged in the conceptual task of developing an ordering system by which the data were organized. The coding system, based on the principles of grounded theory (Strauss & Corbin, 1990), allowed for the generation of themes and a taxonomy of connections among themes, to use for theory-building. Using the transcriptions, two of the primary researchers advanced a process of reading and (re) reading transcripts to develop themes or meaning categories. Each of these researchers read transcripts independently to identify units of analysis for coding purposes. Then, the researchers met to compare and contrast the identified units and to achieve agreement on them. As additional transcripts were reviewed, coding units were added, combined, and clarified. These units were input into the data analysis program and became the base for theory generation. The third primary researcher served as a data consultant at this stage of analysis. This researcher reviewed the coding of the other two researchers and assisted in categorizing of themes and the taxonomy of connections of themes. This approach allowed the three authors to uncover and describe properties of the poorly understood phenomena (Anastas & MacDonald, 1994) of the complex experience of abuse among women with disabilities. The narrative descriptions of the experiences of the participants permitted the emergence of concepts and theoretical tenets that build on previous work.

Participants

All focus group participants were volunteers. Participants were recruited through the Center for Independent Living (CIL) and related

TABLE 1. Participant Characteristics

Group	Number of Males and Females	Disabled	Abuse Survivors[a]	Disability Service Recipient	Disability or Medical Service Provider	Domestic Violence Service Provider	Domestic Violence Service Recipient
1	10 women	9[b]	9	6	4		2
2	5 women 1 man	4[c]	4		5	1	
3	4 women 1 man	4[d]	2		3	1	
4	2 women 1 man	3[e]	3	1	1	1	

a = Indicated that they had been abused in a relationship either in childhood, as an adult, or both.

b = 1 person with Cerebral Palsy, 1 person with Multiple Sclerosis, 1 person with Spina Bifida, 1 person with a degenerative neuromuscular disease, 1 who was a stroke survivor; 2 people had multiple disabilities (one with a brain injury and an undisclosed physical disability, and the other with Multiple Sclerosis and a visual impairment); 1 person with a sensory disability (visual impairment); and 1 person with a learning disability.

c = 1 person who was hard-of-hearing, 1 person with spinal cord injury, 1 who was a stroke survivor, 1 person with a neurological disability.

d = 1 person who was hard-of-hearing and has diabetes and narcolepsy; 2 persons with visual disabilities; and 1 person with spinal muscular atrophy, arthritis, and chronic pain.

e = 1 person who was hard-of-hearing, 1 person who was hard-of-hearing and indicated other disabilities that were not specifically identified to the researchers, 1 person with a muscular skeletal disability and a speech impairment.

disability advocacy organizations in their region. Initial telephone contact to the Executive Directors at each CIL and the designated advocacy organization was made by one of the primary investigators. Participants from a population of physically disabled or nondisabled individuals with a history of or interest in abuse of women with disabilities were recruited for the study. Flyers with information, including telephone numbers for the primary researchers, were posted at the CIL by staff, and forwarded to disability and domestic violence service providers in their areas.

There were 24 participants altogether in the four focus groups. The majority of participants were female, and all but four of the participants identified as having a disability. Seventy-one percent of the participants were professionals, most in the disability or domestic violence fields. Three-quarters of the participants reported that they had been abused as a child and/or adult. Please see Table 1 for more information about participant characteristics.

RESULTS AND DISCUSSION

In analyzing the data, it became clear that the participants reinforced the tenets discussed in the literature review and in previous research. Thus the findings from this study clearly build upon current literature to illuminate the complexity of abuse specific to women with disabilities.

Two major themes embedded within a theoretical structure emerged in data analysis. The themes, discussed below, are: vulnerable beginnings and complexity of abuse. Within the overarching theme of complexity of abuse, three sub-themes were revealed: active abuse, abuse through image, and contextual abuse by social service/legislative systems.

Vulnerable Beginnings

This theme refers to the women's inherent vulnerability that results from being disabled notwithstanding any experience of abuse. Parallel to the experience of adults, who have been sexually abused as children, the informants described the self-depreciation and devaluation that occurs as a common correlate of disablement in and of itself. This phenomenon sets the foundation for exquisite vulnerability to various and complex forms of abuse and for subsequent lack of self-protection.

As stated by one informant,

> Either because of their background, it looks like the women who have been sexually abused as kids get abused in other ways as adults because they have decided that they are dirty, bad or not worth anything. I think in some ways disabled people feel exactly the same thing.

With the backdrop of such low esteem and lack of worth, the complex forms of abuse experienced by disabled women frequently not only occur but often go either unnoticed or unproclaimed by the women themselves.

Complexity of Abuse

The data generated in this study revealed that abuse of women with disabilities is a complex set of structures, tacit meanings, cultural and social assumptions, and systemic service and legislative phenomena. Three sub-thematic levels of abuse emerged in this theme: active abuse, abuse through image, and abuse by contextual social service/legislative systems.

Active Abuse. In concert with previous findings, active abuse perpetrated against women with disabilities occurs in many forms that are not common to nondisabled women. One informant clearly depicted active abuse as follows: "Someone does something that takes advantage of my disability and makes me more disabled than I have to be." This definition clearly shows the placement of disability in the abuse of disabled women.

Illuminating this definition, informants revealed that abuse occurs in many forms. Among them are withholding care; dehumanizing a woman using the disability as the target; refusing to provide care in the manner in which the woman prefers to receive it; using children as leverage to keep a disabled woman in an abusive environment; isolating women with disabilities from support and services; and causing further disablement, illness, and even death through delaying needed care.

One informant states, "So they don't think it's abuse that they are lying in bed all day that they can't even get personal care to come in and help them." Another informant discussed a situation in which the death of a disabled woman could have been prevented by taking her to the emergency room when she needed intervention. As explained by another informant who addresses the complexity of active abuse, "it's not just withholding . . . it's not just throwing out medicine . . . [it's] withholding connection. You know, withholding. I can still give you your pill and dinner but there can be a wall so I am not there, and I will not engage with you at all."

Active abuse also occurs in tacit and hidden forms. Intrusion as a form of unwanted control was frequently revealed as abusive. One informant described the experience of a woman with traumatic brain injury,

> Her mother was intrusive in every aspect of her life down to the time of the day she went to the bathroom and she made her use a scooter indoors, although she could have used a wheelchair or walker, and when she ran into the wall, her mother would scold her very terribly and even in front of me . . . and I thought if she did that in front of me, what is she doing when I'm not there?

Another informant details her experience of intrusion as,

> they carry on . . . and if I happen to be in the way, they casually come over and move my chair out of the way with me in it.

Of particular note is the exploitation of disability accommodations by nondisabled individuals. Several informants indicated that disabled parking placards were taken and used by nondisabled family and friends. One informant related how her nondisabled driver used the informant's disability as an excuse to cancel a parking violation, even though the disabled woman had not been in the car when the violation occurred.

Finally, informants frequently mentioned that active abuse is often a blurring of physical and emotional perpetration. For example, even in the absence of actual physical assault or neglect, the fear of not having basic physical needs addressed because of withholding of assistance is a powerful method by which women with disabilities have been victimized.

Abuse Through Image. This sub-theme refers to abuse occurring as a result of myths, stereotypes, ignorance, and negative attitudes about women with disabilities. Providers as well as family members and other support persons are involved in perpetrating this type of abuse. Mostly, abuse through image is unintended but perpetuated by cultural and social myth about disability.

Many of the informants discussed their experience of being disbelieved by providers when they did report abuse.

> I don't think that the public as a whole think about people with disabilities of any sort . . . as being candidates for abuse. It's just not kosher. It's just not right . . . nobody would do that.

The lack of knowledge, preparation for work with, and devaluing of disabled women by service providers was repeatedly discussed in the focus groups. Of particular importance was the common experience among disabled women as being treated as homogenous, with no attempt on the part of providers to assess how functional incapacity creates the opportunistic context for abuse.

One deaf informant described the humiliating experience of having her sense of isolation being attributed to her disability rather than to the unwillingness of others to accommodate for her communication needs. Other physically disabled informants reported the recurring experience of having abusive situations denied by providers who did not understand the complex interplay of incapacity and caregiver neglect or withholding. Several informants indicated that no one ever asked them about how abuse may have been related to functional incapacity. Another informant with a mental health disability told of providers attributing, without investigation, her report of abuse to the informant's own hallucinations.

The themes of contextual abuse by social service/legislative systems reveals the interactive nature of negative images and large social and cultural systems.

Contextual Abuse by Social Service/Legislative Systems. Informants frequently reported unresponsive, discriminatory and punitive services and legislation as a systemic form of abuse. Despite the passage of protective legislation, the transcripts were replete with descriptions of abusive systems. The negative images described above are carried over in policy and services with the result that systems to identify, document, and intervene in abuse of women with disabilities are not in place. As indicated by one informant in her discussion of her experiences with health and human service agencies,

> I would say to agencies, I realize I have a disability and that my disability is not so much what is supposedly wrong with me but I find my disability is more your attitude about what is wrong with me . . . if you would just put your attitude aside and help me, I'd appreciate that greatly.

Systemic abuse includes limited or absent access to resources that are available to nondisabled abused women, such as shelters, knowledgeable providers, and targeted protective legislation against the unique abuse experienced by disabled women. One informant stated that she was unlikely to report abuse for fear of losing care assistance from providers who declared that they would refer her elsewhere for all services if she required abuse protection. Other informants were referred to rehabilitation units or accessible medical environments when they called community shelters for protection. Systemic abuse perpetuates a context in which active abuse by image can continue.

Finally, to complete the analysis, a summary statement emerged from the transcripts which provides a basic theoretical taxonomy for abuse of disabled women. An informant identified abuse as a continuing social/cultural paradox between social sanction of caregiving based on functional incapacity and social devaluation of women with disabilities. That is to say, while the obligation for care is apparent and paid to a certain extent by social supports, this care is "bestowed" on socially and culturally devalued women with disabling conditions. Continuing from the discourse of the informant quoted directly above is a clear plea: "just acknowledge me as a human being, as a woman." Continued devaluation perpetuates the continuation of unresponsive systems and services, as well as the exclusion of disabled women from the mainstream of abuse services.

CONCLUSIONS

These data present a clear image of the complexity of abuse of women with disabilities. From the data analysis, important theory has been suggested for future testing and verification. Yet the findings also provide current direction to inform curriculum and practice.

First and most critical is the recognition that the experience of disability in and of itself creates vulnerability to victimization as well as the potential to amplify abusive acts if they should occur. Given the existence of an already vulnerable position, it is clear that abused, disabled women, although holding significant commonalties with abused nondisabled women, are distinct and unique, thereby equiring targeted research and provider training. As indicated in previous research (Gilson et al., in press), actions that may seem non-threatening to nondisabled women, may not only be harmful but can be life threatening to women with disabilities. Withholding and/or neglect are serious and potentially abusive to women who cannot provide care for themselves due to functional incapacity. Moreover, tacit, hidden, or unintended actions can be seriously harmful to disabled women who cannot counter such assaults or who cannot garner assistance in doing so.

Further adding to the complexity of abuse of disabled women is the notion of abuse as image. As described in detail above, image itself is multifaceted and provides the context for the continuation of individual, family, community, service, legislative, and cultural unresponsiveness to abused women with disabilities. While many disenfranchised groups experience these oppressive phenomena, what expands negative image from oppression to abuse in disabled women is the extensive physical and emotional harm that results from only seeing an individual as her intrinsic disabling condition rather than as a member of a vulnerable cultural/social group in need of responsive and protective services. Shortsightedness as a function of negative image places the full burden for tolerance of or emergence from abusive situations clearly on the disabled individual who, if she even ventures to seek help, is referred to services which sublimate harmful social circumstances to a system which devotes its effort to curing individual deficits. Moreover, traditional systems serving disabled individuals have placed care receivers in a devalued role in which provision of care is seen not as civil right but as charity. This paternalistic perspective perpetuates silence, powerlessness, and continued exposure to abuse in disabled women who are expected to be thankful for care. While being expected to be grateful for the care bestowed upon them, disabled women are also taught to not question or challenge the manner in which the care is provided, thus learned compliance is enforced (Chenoweth, 1996).

In extending the traditional definition of abuse to image, theorists, researchers, and practitioners need to examine and attend to the contextual nature of abuse, and address its differential and unique appearance in diverse populations. Advancing contextual definitions of abuse is incumbent on theorists, providers, and researchers to assure that abuse is not neglected or overlooked for all victims because of conceptual monism.

Building on the notion of heterogeneity of the nature of abuse, of particular importance is the homogenization of disabled women and the failure on the part of theory to provide assessment and practice guidance. As revealed by the data, the interplay of functional incapacity and abuse is a critical tenet to be tested and attended to in any effort to address and mediate abuse of women with diverse disabilities.

Regardless of the condition, abuse of disabled women is both influenced by and affects the ability to carry out activities of daily living (ADLs) and instrumental activities of daily living (IADLs). Activities of daily living include those associated with toileting, eating, transferring into or out of a bed or chair, dressing, taking a bath or shower, and getting around inside the home. Instrumental activities of daily living include those such as attending school, shopping, working, participation in community activities, preparing meals, using the telephone, doing light housework, and keeping track of money and bills.

IMPLICATIONS

This research has important implications for future research and for current curriculum development and practice. Future research with large and diverse samples of disabled women should be conducted to test, revise and codify theory for use. However, the cumulative knowledge generated by both the study conducted herein and previous studies suggests important direction for curriculum and practice. Curriculum can be informed by distinguishing environmental and individual contexts for abuse and intervention. Students can be introduced to the diversity of abuse and its correlates and to the critical need to develop targeted, responsive practices. Of particular note is the need to establish assessment procedures that can identify abuse in the diverse population of disabled women. Key to this identification is the recognition that assessment of individual function in ADLs and IADLs is essential in any assessment of abuse in disabled women. Assessment of functional capacity not only can reveal areas of vulnerability, but can reveal functional strengths which cannot be exercised by women because they are being limited by abuse rather than disability.

Limitations for the present study include the self-selection process of the participants, wherein the population does not reflect the heterogeneity of the disability community. Although a strength of the study was the mix of service providers and service recipients, this could have served to inhibit the full disclosure and discussion by those individuals receiving services. Additionally, the time limit of the focus group format may have served to provide arbitrary closure to the group process.

Scholars, students, and practitioners will be better able to serve this vulnerable, oppressed, and underserved population if empirical inquiry continues to elucidate the experiences, service and support needs, and the system's change needs of abused women with disabilities.

Finally, this study has important implications for understanding human behavior and advancing human behavior theory in a broad sense. Because theory is an attempt to explain and predict phenomena, it speaks to generalities and provides a road map, so to speak, for understanding. And while maps provide critical guidelines, they miss the nuances and dimensions necessary for fully informed and successful navigation. Building on the vast body of literature on human diversity, this inquiry reminds us that theoretical maps must be synthesized with unique individual and contextual phenomena in order to capture the complexity, breadth, and depth of human experience and need. Thus, both nomothetic and idiographic understandings of humans are essential in elucidating human behavior theory and knowledge to inform policy, practice, and social change efforts.

NOTE

1. The terms women with disabilities and disabled women are used interchangeably. This mixed use reflects the current thinking on the use of language by, among, and with individuals with disabilities. Please see and Gilson, Tusler, & Gill (1997); Heumann (1993); among others.

REFERENCES

Anastas, J. W., & MacDonald, M. L. (1994). *Research design for social work and the human services.* New York, NY: Lexington.

Barnes, C., & Mercer, G. (1997). *Doing disability research.* Leeds, England: Disability Press.

Berkeley Planning Associates. (1992). *Meeting the needs of women with disabilities: A blueprint for change.* Berkeley, CA: Author.

Calvey, P. (1998, July). *The invisible woman: Women with disabilities and abuse.* Paper presented at the 8th National Conference & 20-Year Anniversary, National Coalition Against Domestic Violence, Denver, CO.

Chenoweth, L. (1996). Violence and women with disabilities. *Violence Against Women, 2*(4), 391-411.

Creswell, J. W. (1994). *Research design: Quantitative and qualitative approaches.* Thousand Oaks, CA: Sage.

DePoy, E., & Gitlin, L. (1998). *Introduction to research: Understanding and applying multiple methods.* St. Louis, MO: Mosby.

Frey, J. H., & Fontana, A. (1993). The group interview in social research. In David L. Morgan (Ed.), *Successful focus groups: Advancing the state of the art* (pp. 20-34). Newbury Park, CA: Sage.

Gill, C. J., Kirschner, K. L., & Panko Reis, J. (1994). Health services for women with disabilities: Barriers and portals. In A. Dun (Ed.). *Referring women's health: Multidisciplinary research and practice* (pp. 357-366). Thousand Oaks, CA: Sage.

Gilson, S. F., Cramer, E. P., & DePoy, E. (in press). (Re)Defining abuse of women with disabilities: A paradox of limitation and expansion. *AFFILIA: Journal of Women and Social Work.*

Gilson, S. F., Tusler, A., & Gill, C. J. (1997). Ethnographic research in disability identity: Self-determination and community. *Journal of Vocational Rehabilitation, 9,* 7-17.

Heumann, J. E. (1993). Building our own boats: A personal perspective on disability. In L. O. Gostin & H. A. Beyer (Eds.), *Implementing the Americans with Disabilities Act: Rights and responsibilities of all Americans* (pp. 251-263). Baltimore: Paul H. Brookes.

National Coalition Against Domestic Violence. (1996). *Open minds, open doors.* Denver, CO: Author.

Nosek, M. A., Rintala, D. H., Young, M. E., Foley, C. C., Howland, C., Chanpong, G. F., Rossi, D., Bennett, J., & Meroney, K. (undated). *National study of women with physical disabilities: Special summary.* Houston, TX: Center for Research on Women with Disabilities.

QSR NUD*IST (version 4.0) [computer software]. (1996). Thousand Oaks, CA: Sage Publications Software.

Reinharz, S. (1992). *Feminist methods in social research.* New York: Oxford University Press.

Seelman, K. D., & Sweeney, S. M. (1997). Empowerment, advocacy, and self-determination: Initiatives of the National Institute on Disability and Rehabilitation Research. *Journal of Vocational Rehabilitation, 9,* 65-71.

Sobsey, R. (1994). *Violence in the lives of people with disabilities: The end of silent acceptance?* Baltimore, MD: Brookes.

Strauss, A., & Corbin, J. (1990). *Basics of qualitative research: Grounded theory procedures and techniques.* Newbury Park, CA: Sage.

Tjaden, P., & Thoennes, N. (1998, November). *Prevalence, incidence, and consequences of violence against women: Findings from the National Violence Against Women Survey. Research in brief.* National Institute of Justice. Centers for Disease Control.

Young, M. E., Nosek, M. A., Howland, C., Chanpong, G., & Rintala, D. H. (1997). Prevalence of abuse of women with physical disabilities. *Archives of Physical Medicine and Rehabilitation, 78,* Suppl. 5, S34-S38.

Caregiving Issues for Grandmothers Raising Their Grandchildren

Deborah P. Waldrop

SUMMARY. Increasing numbers of middle aged and older adults are raising their grandchildren as a result of complex family problems, and a majority of these caregivers are women. Precipitating problems such as drug
abuse, child neglect or parental incarceration are difficult social problems
that cause unique caregiving problems for grandparents who step in to stabilize a chaotic family situation. In-depth interviews were conducted with 37
women who were raising grandchildren. Results indicate that grandmothers
who raise their grandchildren experience both burdens and benefits from
their roles as family caregivers. Increased understanding about the special
needs and problems of this group of family caregivers will enhance practice
effectiveness with these multi-generational families. *[Article copies available
for a fee from The Haworth Document Delivery Service: 1-800-HAWORTH.
E-mail address: <docdelivery@haworthpress.com> Website: <http://www.
HaworthPress.com> © 2003 by The Haworth Press, Inc. All rights reserved.]*

KEYWORDS. Grandmothers raising grandchildren, grandparent
caregiving, family stress

Deborah P. Waldrop, CSW, PhD, is Assistant Professor, School of Social Work,
University at Buffalo, 630 Baldy Hall, Box 601050, Buffalo, NY 14260-1050 (Email:
dwaldrop@acsu.buffalo.edu).

[Haworth co-indexing entry note]: "Caregiving Issues for Grandmothers Raising Their Grandchildren."
Waldrop, Deborah P. Co-published simultaneously in *Journal of Human Behavior in the Social Environment*
(The Haworth Social Work Practice Press, an imprint of The Haworth Press, Inc.) Vol. 7, No. 3/4, 2003,
pp. 201-223; and: *Women and Girls in the Social Environment: Behavioral Perspectives* (ed: Nancy J. Smyth)
The Haworth Social Work Practice Press, an imprint of The Haworth Press, Inc., 2003, pp. 201-223. Single or
multiple copies of this article are available for a fee from The Haworth Document Delivery Service
[1-800-HAWORTH, 9:00 a.m. - 5:00 p.m. (EST). E-mail address: docdelivery@haworthpress.com].

Digital Object Identifier: 10.1300/J137v7n03_12

Caregivers play critical family roles as they helping vulnerable and dependent loved ones who need assistance with activities of every day life. Historically, caregiving research has focused on the needs of people with a particular physical illness or disability such as Alzheimer's disease (Biegel & Shulz, 1999). The phrase "family caregiving" has most often been used to describe informal help, which is provided for an older adult in deteriorating health. Daughters and daughters-in-law have been most well known as family caregivers (Baum & Page, 1991). More recent research efforts have viewed the essential function of family caregiving through a broader lens, which includes others such as parents of disabled adults and grandparents raising grandchildren (Kaufman, 1998; Lefley, 1996; Roe & Minkler, 1998). Researchers have begun to consider both the similarities and differences among diverse groups of caregivers and to explore their unique issues. This broader focus enhances understanding of the needs of previously marginalized populations (Minkler & Roe, 1993; Strawbridge, Wallhagen, Shema, & Kaplan, 1997).

The provision of ongoing assistance to a dependent person changes the life of a caregiver. Historically, caregiving has been seen as burdensome to the extent that the responsibility infringes upon an individual's life (Brody, 1981; Zarit, Reever, & Bach-Peterson, 1980). More recently, studies have described psychological gains that come from caregiving relationships (Kramer, 1997; Ryff, 1989). Positive outcomes emerge from facing the challenges of family problems within the context of close relationships. Accomplishment on behalf of another can create new meaning in an individual's life.

This paper will explore the unique family caregiving issues of grandmothers who are raising grandchildren. It will examine both the positive and negative outcomes of caregiving for women in this situation. Participants' words and stories will be used to illustrate the manner in which grandparents' issues are similar and different to caregiving in other family situations.

FAMILY CAREGIVING

Caring is an essential component of close relationships. Chronic or progressive impairment changes a close relationship by forcing caregiving to become the focus of interaction. Caregiving is articulated as an extension of the essential qualities of ongoing family relationships (Pearlin, Mullan, Semple, & Skaff, 1990). The need for family caregiving can also result from non-normative family events. Regardless of the etiology, the tasks of caring can range from minimal and infrequent to intense and frequent.

Informal care has been characterized to include the everyday activities of managing a household or performing personal care such as dressing, bathing, toileting and feeding, which is provided by family and friends (National Alliance for Caregiving, 1997). The intensity, with which some or all of these tasks are completed, varies widely among situations and depends on the person's needs. Formal care is characterized as the assistance of a paid caregiver or from a professional homecare agency. Family caregivers who provide informal care often find support from the formal system, which maintains stability and diminishes burden (Auslander & Litwin, 1995). While caregiving appears to add new burdens to otherwise normal lives for spouse and adult-child caregivers, it becomes yet another aspect of a difficult life course for grandparent caregivers (Minkler & Roe, 1993; Strawbridge et al., 1997).

Family stress theory provides the theoretical framework that guides this study. The concepts of stressors, coping mechanisms, and adaptation found in family stress theory are consistently used in caregiving research. Studies about caregiving have considered the contribution of the social context, tasks performed, secondary role strain, and family resources as conceptualized by Pearlin, Mullan, Semple, and Skaff (1990). Stressors for grandparents raising their grandchildren arise from individual, family, and community problems faced by grandparents in this situation (Burnette, 1999a; Burton, 1992). Grandparents raising their grandchildren face emotional, family, financial, social, and legal health challenges.

PROFILES OF FAMILY CAREGIVERS

The prevalence of family caregiving is becoming more widely recognized. Recently established, the National Alliance for Caregiving (1997) estimates that there are more than 22 million households providing care to a relative or friend who is aged 50 or older. Caregiving, which is rendered to older dependent family members, most often evolves gradually and over time. Caregiving tasks evolve from a relationship in which many different needs are met. Parent care is considered both a normative stress and filial obligation (Brody, 1981), but the necessity for family caregiving in grandparent headed households results from non-normative family events.

Disruptive family problems, which are precipitated by the drug abuse, child neglect or death of an adult child, force grandparent caregivers to begin juggling the roles of grandparent and parent simultaneously. Grandparent caregivers forge new roles for themselves by facing multiple challenges, which require strength, creativity, and determination. The 1990 census highlighted a forty-four percent (44%) increase of children who are being raised by grandparents during the past decade. Current estimates indicate that nearly four million American children now live in households headed by grandparents (Fuller-Thomson, Minkler, & Driver, 1997; Lugaila, 1999).

Studies demonstrate that women provide more dependent care than men do (Kramer, 1997). Seventy-three percent (73%) of the caregivers for older adults are female. The profile is further characterized as married women in their mid-forties, sixty-four percent (64%) of whom balance work and caregiving obligations (National Alliance on Caregiving, 1997). The national profile of grandparent caregivers is also primarily female and further specified as maternal grandmothers who are African-American and living in the inner city (Fuller-Thompson, Minkler, & Driver, 1997). Most caregivers willingly accept the challenges and responsibilities they face despite the associated hardships.

CONSEQUENCES OF CAREGIVING

Many early studies focused on the negative outcomes of providing care for a dependent person (Kramer, 1997; Ryff, 1989). Caregiver burden was conceptualized as psychological distress, anxiety, depression, and generalized loss of personal freedom resulting from the responsibility for total care of another individual (Pruchno, Burant, & Peters, 1997; Zarit et al., 1980). Burden is the extent to which a caregiver experiences physical, social, mental, or spiritual suffering which results from providing care for a family member. Caregiver burden is also equated with strain in secondary roles that are affected by the provision of care for a dependent person. Women provide more intensive types of care and experience more secondary role strains than men do. They are also more likely to experience higher levels of burden and work-role strains (Kramer & Kipnis, 1995).

The relationship between caregiving and well-being has been conceptualized as having both positive and negative effects (Kramer, 1997; Ryff, 1989). Ryff (1989) developed six distinct dimensions of well-being that offer balance to the field of caregiving. The positive elements of caregiving include personal growth, purpose in life, autonomy, environmental mastery, positive relations with others, and self-acceptance (Ryff, 1989). The caregiver gains self-confidence and personal gratification from managing the crisis. This perspective challenges researchers to consider both positive and negative effects of grandparent caregiving.

Dimensions of the Caregiving Experience

The stress of caregiving has been well documented (Kramer, 1997; Pearlin et al., 1990; Pruchno et al., 1997). Caregiver stress is found to result from extraordinary and unequally distributed burden (Pearlin et al., 1990). Research literature portrays caregiving most often as burdensome and negative. Previous research in family caregiving has described four dimensions of the caregiving experience, which are salient in the exploration of grandparent caregiving (Sharlach, 1994): ongoing family relationships, work and family responsibilities, emotional and psychological responses, and health.

Ongoing Family Relationships

Throughout the life course, family members care for one another, return favors, and depend on each other for assistance. Informal support is a regular part of family interactions. The relationship between a family caregiver and someone who is chronically ill reflects previous aspects of the relationship as well as different boundaries, which change with increased dependence (Biegel & Shulz, 1999; Thiede-Call, Finch, Huck, & Kane, 1999). A parent's chronic illness may precipitate the need for an adult child caregiver to begin bathing a parent or managing his or her personal finances. Family relationships are changed by the events, which precipitate caregiving and continue evolving over time.

Grandparent caregiving follows an event or series of difficult and stressful events. Consequently, these family problems change the sequences of the normative stages of family development. Middle-aged and older adults begin parenting their grandchildren with added difficulties which are related to the children's traumatic experiences. Children who have been exposed to cocaine, alcohol, or HIV/AIDS before birth often have complications. Children who have been abused and traumatized by a parent's actions may have behavioral outbursts. Poverty exacerbates problems by limiting the resources, which can be applied to such complex issues (Burton, 1992; Joslin & Brouard, 1995). The developmental tasks that ordinarily accompany grandparenting are diminished by the magnitude of the family problems. The experiences of grandparent caregivers are different than those faced by others in the same age cohort.

Work-Family Responsibilities

Simultaneous family and work responsibilities create pressures, which affect caregivers' well-being. Work and family roles compete for available time and energy. The responsibilities of conflicting roles make caregivers especially vulnerable to stress related health problems (Shulz & Beach, 1999). The National Alliance on Caregiving describes the intersection between work and family responsibilities for individuals to include juggling competing demands, lost or changed career opportunities, and substantial financial impact from caregiving expenses (National Alliance for Caregiving, 1999). Grandmother caregivers indicated they had work-related problems such as lateness or missed days because they were dealing with a grandchild or they changed the number of hours to accommodate the child (Pruchno, 1999).

Emotional and Psychological Reactions

Family caregiving involves intense emotional and psychological reactions. Emotions can simultaneously involve both positive and negative feelings. Joy and satisfaction or anger and fear can coexist. Caregiving is "emotion work," and an inability to manage the intense, associated feelings may well be a very important component of caregiver stress (McRae, 1998). Caregiver stress results from extraordinary and unequally distributed burden (Pearlin et al., 1990). Nevertheless, research literature portrays caregiving most often as burdensome and negative.

Health Issues

Grandparents involved in raising their grandchildren experience stressors that can potentially affect their physical health. Roe, Minkler, Saunders, and Thomson (1996) evaluated self-reported health status. Participants reported good physical health with little change since caregiving began but they do not see physicians regularly. There is an important distinction to be made between denial of symptoms and reframing an illness to manage the routine of daily life. Roe et al. (1996) speculate that grandparent caregivers often reframe their symptoms to gain a sense of control in the situation. Grandparent caregivers are thought to be hidden patients, potentially at risk for health problems themselves (Roe et al., 1996). It is possible that grandparent caregivers may use denial or minimization of physical symptoms as a method of functioning in this difficult situation.

The purpose of this study was to compare the caregiving experiences of grandmothers who are raising their grandchildren with those of other family caregivers. The dimensions of ongoing relationships, work-family intersection, emotional and psychological reactions, and health issues were explored with grandmother caregivers.

METHODOLOGY

This qualitative study was exploratory and descriptive in nature. It was part of a larger study on grandparent-headed households which employed semi-structured in-depth interviews that were conducted with 37 women who were primary caregivers for one or more grandchildren. The focus of the study was to explore specific caregiving issues related for grandmothers in this situation. The study took place in a midwestern state and participants lived in a wide geographic area including both urban and rural areas.

Sample

Grandmother participants ranged in age from 41-76 with the mean age being 56.4 years. Most of the informants were married. Fifteen participants were in original marriages and raising the grandchildren of both spouses. Thirteen were raising their grandchild(ren) with a second husband. The study population was primarily white, although it included two African American and one Native American grandmother caregivers. The sample was comprised of nearly equal groups who lived in metropolitan areas, small towns and in rural, farming communities. Recruitment of participants occurred in several ways. Grandparents who had attended a statewide conference for caregivers or attended a local support group were invited to participate. A snowball effect occurred as grandparents led the researcher to other caregivers they knew.

Grandmother participants were raising a total of sixty-one children. More women were raising a daughter's children than were raising a son's children, and two were raising children from both a son and daughter. The children's ages range from 6 months to 22 years. Three families included young adults who were raised by grandparents and were in college or living independently. Grandparent participants included these young adults when they described the grandchildren they were raising. Table 1 illustrates the demographics of grandmother caregivers in this sample.

Interviews

The interviews were guided by the use of an instrument, which had open-ended questions. The instrument was adapted from that used by Minkler and Roe (1993) in their initial study of grandmother caregivers. Additional questions about health, financial, legal, social, and emotional issues, as well as coping mechanisms were added. Individual interviews were scheduled in a location chosen by participants and proceeded at a pace and direction they established. Interview locations included the participants' homes, restaurants, or places of employment. All but one of the participants allowed the researcher to audiotape the interviews, and tapes were later transcribed.

RESULTS AND ANALYSIS

Data analysis was twofold. First, response typologies were created for answers to structured questions. Second, participants' stories were reviewed and analyzed for common themes, which occurred across interviews. Interview transcripts were coded by using QSR NUD*IST software. QSR NUD*IST software allowed the establishment of pre-existing and new or "free" categories. The use of free categories facilitated the discovery of themes, which emerged from interview data. Frequency counts were compiled for themes that emerged. Participants often gave more than one answer, so counts do not add to one hundred percent (100%).

Four dimensions of the caregiving experience, (1) ongoing-family relationships, (2) work-family responsibilities, (3) emotional and psychological reactions, and (4) health, served as categories for coding. Sections about these four dimensions describe the responses, which emerged as themes from interview data in two ways. Frequency counts illustrate the response typologies, and participants' words and anecdotes further portray their experiences. The fifth section, (5) strength in adversity, describes a new theme that emerged from interviews with grandmother caregivers.

TABLE 1. Demographic Characteristics of Grandparent Caregivers (n = 37)

Categories	Number	Percent
Marital Status:		
Widowed	5	11%
Divorced	4	14%
Married	46	75%
Original marriage	15	40%
Step-family	12	35%
Whose children raising?		
Daughter's children	22	59%
Raising son's children	13	36%
Raising children of more than one family member	2	5%
Occupational Status		
Employed full time outside of the home	15	41%
Employed, working at home	5	14%
Full time students	3	8%
Retired	6	16%
Not employed at this time	8	22%
Number of Grandchildren Raising		
1	23	61%
2	8	21%
3	6	16%
4	1	3%
Length of time raising grandchildren:		
≤ 1 year	10	16%
1-5 years	28	44%
6-10 years	14	22%
11-15 years	5	7%
>15 years	7	11%

Ongoing Family Relationships

Ongoing family relationships are a constant concern for grandmothers who are raising their grandchildren. Despite efforts to stabilize the situation, grandparents continue to worry about problems in their families. The dramatic problems, which cause an adult child's inability to function as a parent, are an underlying concern for their mothers. Grandmothers also expressed continuing concern about grandchildren's well being.

Grandmothers were asked about the greatest sources of stress in their lives. Family relationships were the primary concern in all situations. Forty-three percent (43%) of the participants identified the greatest source of stress as their grandchild(ren)'s well being. Thirty-five (35%) of the participants explained that their adult child's well being caused the most stress for them.

One 49-year-old grandmother described her concerns about a grandchild who had been court ordered to visit her mother on a weekly basis, in this way:

> Here is this precious 11-year-old girl who laid in her bed and said, Grammy, I would rather be dead than to have to go back to her (mother's) house tomorrow. It absolutely broke my heart. I know her momma was mean to her and beat her and it is not right that she has to go back there.

Grandmothers also expressed grave concerns that their children would further harm a grandchild. The words of a 46-year-old grandmother illustrate concern about her grandson's safety:

> I am extremely protective of Neal (her 5-year-old grandson) because I am always afraid of her (his mother). It is real spooky, I have to live on the edge, because I never know what she or that crowd is going to do and I worry that she will kidnap him (from school). I feel like I always have to watch out and that makes me so angry.

Grandmothers expressed profound concerns about their adult child. Participants gave detailed descriptions of the efforts they had made to help an adult child, and of deep disappointment that their efforts had not succeeded. They described ongoing stress about the well-being and life style of a troubled adult child. Some adult children were actively using drugs and had episodic eruptions of criminal, erratic or abusive behavior. Grandparents described fear about their adult child's lifestyle and continued concern that harm or death would result from a drug habit or from their unsavory associates.

One 48-year-old grandmother describes her manner of coping with her daughter's ongoing drug use in this way:

She was here at Christmas and I told her that her biggest present for me this year was letting her go. I still love her and I'm still her mom. I'm still delighted that she calls and I would love for her to come over if she calls and makes arrangements. We never allow her to drop in because I need to make sure she's not using, but I just have ceased expectations. I'm not putting any pressure on her to do anything anymore. She took it like I was breaking up with her. Today's her birthday and that's difficult. I didn't break up with her; I just let her go. There's a big difference.

Other participants expressed the profound loss they have felt about their adult child's inability to change, and the resulting fear they live with daily. This grandmother's words express this fear:

My daughter disappears and I don't know if I'll ever see her again. I realize now that we could give her everything we have and she would still be using. I've told her I would give my life if it would make her stop.

Another participant further describes ongoing stress in this way:

I don't know if most people feel this way but when you have a 16-year-old daughter on the street, it is better to imagine her dead than to imagine all the things that could be happening to her. She would be better of dead than doing the things I could imagine. I wanted to be hopeful but my imagination wouldn't let me. I imagined her dead in those years, many times, and truthfully, dead is better than what I could have imagined.

Most participants expressed feelings of helplessness about how the relationship with their adult child had gotten out of control. This 55-year-old grandmother's words express that feeling:

I really don't understand how it happened. Sometimes I look at her and wonder what went wrong.

Many participants also described ongoing family relationships in a positive light. One 53-year-old grandmother who was raising a 7-year-old described joy she feels in raising her grandson:

> I think of the joy often because, well probably because there was so many times that I had to remind myself that there was joy, but he is absolutely a joy, and I've always known this–I knew this with my own children, if you love a child they will love you so completely back and they are so trusting of you, and I you know like I said I felt that way with my own children and I've really, really enjoyed for the most part having Tommy, I enjoyed him even as a baby and holding him and, and being home with him which I was not able to do with my children, I mean I was at home with them but I was working and cleaning house and you know all the other things I thought I had to do that I don't think that I have to do anymore you know. But I would definitely to tell others to keep a journal, or meditate, or pray, but you know you've got to acknowledge what you feel, not vent it but acknowledge it yourself and say it okay for me to feel this way.

A 76-year-old grandmother retrospectively discusses the ongoing relationship with her 17-year-old grandson this way:

> I think in realizing we've got him this far. You know. That he has had a much better life than he would have had. One year his mother moved seven times. And you know this she had been pretty stationary, the last two years she'd been in the same place. But he has had a much better life than he would have ever had.

Family relationships continue despite great conflict and struggle. Participants described continuing efforts they made to stabilize the relationship with an adult child and to provide stability for their grandchildren. In essence, grandmothers in this situation are caregivers for both the grandchildren they are raising as well as for their troubled adult children.

Work-Family Responsibilities

Work-family responsibilities were an issue for sixty-eight percent (68%) of the sample. This category includes participants who were employed outside the home (41%), inside the home (14%), or were full-time students (8%). Thirty-two percent (32%) of the sample was retired or presently not employed.

Grandmothers discussed both negative and positive results from balancing work and family responsibilities. Job related issues, finances, and child care were expressed as the primary work related issues that concerned them. Financial strain was further explored, and the greatest source of financial strain resulted from an increased cost of living. In seventeen percent (17%) of the situations, grandmother caregivers felt pressure to work. Six percent (6%) of the participants expressed no additional financial concerns related to raising grandchildren.

Grandmothers expressed concerns about their abilities to find and keep employment at this later time in life. The words of a 53-year-old grandmother express the realities for many:

> And at this time it's kind of hard because we really need the insurance and when you are fifty-three years old and you've had cancer it is kind of hard to change jobs. Even just plain fifty-three they don't want to hire you; you're too old.

Participants who were employed outside of the home discussed the increased stress they felt impacted on their work. This 51-year-old grandmother explained:

> I've worked there for 27 years and I had made it to being a supervisor but I just got to the point where I couldn't take the stress. I cannot take it. So I went back as an hourly person. I am not making as much money as I used to but I work eight hours and go home.

Grandparent caregivers expressed feelings of being trapped in a particular job because it provided stability and economic security. This 59-year-old grandmother's words illustrate:

> Now like I'm saying I love these kids, but if I didn't have the kids I might have quit. I might have just said, I know I can make a living for me somewhere but you know I've got the benefits here, I can get a retirement from here and then I got a lot of money saved up in the credit union and I just bought me this house. I'm gonna be sixty years old soon, and then after two more years I'm gonna try to retire and run a daycare at home.

Participants also expressed positive aspects of balancing work-family responsibilities. This 47-year-old grandmother found a emotional and social support in her work:

> People that I work with are wonderful. They are just marvelous. They work with me, they support me and say, "Sadie is there any-

thing that I can do to help you," and stuff like that. It makes a 100% difference as opposed to people who won't work with you and I've had it both ways. Work is my support. There were times when I worked full-time at the burn center, part time at the hospital, and then I squeezed in a part-time job 1 day per week at the shelter. I refused to get on welfare. I refused food stamps . . . I just worked my butt off.

Other grandparent caregivers were caring for more than one dependent family member and found support at their place of employment. The words of this 54-year-old grandmother who was caring for a husband with dementia and a granddaughter illustrate:

And what's great is that my manager at work and those working with me helped me look at what I am going to do so I can retire, what am I going to do when he (husband) needs help just to stay at home. She kind of reversed that and said what we need to look at is what we can do to keep you on the job. What can we do to help you, keep on working, and insurance benefits for Annie (granddaughter). And that is different from what I was expecting. She gave me different options to look at.

Balancing work and family responsibilities was not a new experience for any of the participants who were employed. Consideration of middle and later life issues made these issues different than at earlier life stages for grandmother caregivers in this study.

Emotional and Psychological Reactions

Grandmothers expressed profound emotional and psychological responses to their experiences as grandparent caregivers. These responses were both negative and positive. Negative feelings included dread, fear, anxiety, and loss, which were primarily related to the adult child's situation. Positive feelings included delight in their grandchild's growth, a sense of accomplishment, and feelings of peace about making a difference in the previously turbulent life of a grandchild. The typology of emotional responses which emerged included feeling well, feelings of anger and resentment, grief, and loss.

Seventeen percent (17%) of the participants expressed feelings of anger and resentment. Grandparents expressed anger that was directed at many sources. Adult children, the legal system, spouses and the social service system were all foci for grandparents' anger.

A 53-year-old grandmother explained:

> When I started raising the girls, my other daughters were having children. Part of me is angry because I never got to be a grandma to Tara and Penny; I was too busy being Mom again.

Forty-six percent (46%) of the participants described feelings of overwhelming loss and grief. Grandparent caregiving involves the loss of hopes and dreams about the future and about an adult child. In some situations there were multiple prior losses, including spouses, siblings and parents. There is also loss of a normative and anticipated grandparent role, which was reinforced daily. Grief was described in every aspect of grandparents' lives.

The words of a 61-year-old grandmother, who lost two sons in drug related deaths, expresses her response to her losses in this way:

> When I was a child, my mother involved herself in a very bad relationship with lots of fighting and I would go to bed and be awakened at night and pray and pray and pray, "Please God make them stop fighting. Please God make them stop fighting." Well when I was a senior in college, Dad died of a heart attack and the conflict had not ceased by then, I mean the thing that ended it was his death. When my boys were in using drugs, I used to pray "Please stop using drugs" Well, Dan did for awhile, and then died. So I can't pray for things like that. What I do believe and what I can pray for is support and comfort and I get that through people and I truly think that God works through people. So in that way religion helps but it's the concrete when to run to another person that sustains me and having friends that I can talk to. I do have kind of a handful of close friends I can talk to about things like this.

Grandparents expressed emotional pain experienced from their adult child's problems. This 47-year-old grandmother who is raising children from both a son and a daughter illustrates:

> When my son was using I worked and tried and helped him. When my 15-year-old became pregnant I was really hurt. I thought she had learned from watching her brother and from watching her step sister who has been pregnant, not educated, and not married. I can

want and want and want for her but if she doesn't want it for herself then it doesn't make any difference.

A small but important seven percent (7%) of the grandparent caregivers described their response as an emotional shutdown. One 50-year-old grandmother who was raising her daughter's three children expressed this response by saying:

> It is awful to say but I don't have any feelings for her. I don't know who she is. I was sick, sick, sick. You know I would be up a lot at night praying out the window and wondering if you know . . . I'd get up in the middle of the night to go drive by and make sure the house wasn't burning down. Then I just shut down; I don't get emotional anymore.

Finally, it is important to note that unconditional parental love was included in many parents' descriptions of their adult child. Despite the emotional upheaval an adult child may have caused, parents expressed their continuing love and hope for that adult child's future. Positive feelings emanated from the accomplishments they felt at providing security and safety for their grandchild(ren) in difficult circumstances. Eleven percent (11%) expressed their overwhelming emotional response to grandparent caregiving as feeling good. Others expressed the joy and delight they felt from watching a grandchild thrive. The words of a 46-year-old grandmother express joy,

> She is so much happiness and such a joy, I am overwhelmed with the blessing that she is. This 4-year-old is so full of life and love, so interesting and it is so wonderful to be around her.

Grandmothers expressed myriad emotions, which were complex and interrelated. Their responses illustrate the profound impact these experiences have on the life of the caregiver.

Health Issues

Grandmothers were asked about whether their health had changed during the time that they had been raising grandchildren. Eighty-nine percent (89%) believed that their health had been affected. Twenty-two percent of the participants felt that caregiving exacerbated pre-existing conditions such as diabetes, hypertension, or cardiac disease. Twenty-four percent (24%) expressed feeling increased fatigue. Sixteen percent (16%) explained that they experienced increased susceptibility to colds and gastric upset. Fourteen percent (14%) were in treatment for depression.

A 48-year-old grandmother raising three grandchildren expresses general fatigue this way:

> I feel twenty years older now because I'm so much more tired. But, I do have a lot more reasons to want to be healthy.

A 55-year-old grandmother expresses the connection she sees between stress and health in these words:

> You're more prone to illness when you're stressed. And you see in the last five years my father died of AIDS, my father-in-law died of cancer and in between our fathers passing away we've lost two uncles and an aunt and our other son and his wife and child were staying with us, her brother had a fire in their house and two children died there. My best friend in high school and her husband were murdered, and my boss's seven-year-old daughter died of a heart attack. My husband lost his job and had a stroke. And we've been trying to deal with all this stuff with Andy.

Eleven percent of the participants believed that their health had not been affected by the grandparent caregiving, or that their problems were age related rather than caregiving related. One 60-year-old grandmother illustrates this by saying,

> What happened to my health was going to happen anyway. I have very bad knees. It is hard to keep up the energy level I need, I just wish I had more energy.

A small but notable eight percent (8%) explained that they believe that caregiving had actually improved their health status. These participants explained that they had become more active because they were raising grandchildren.

Strength in Adversity

Grandmother caregivers discussed the difficulties they had experienced in both dealing with a troubled adult child and in beginning to parent young children again. An important theme of strength in adversity was discussed by seventeen percent (17%) of grandmother caregivers. Grandmothers explained that handling the challenges of a troubled adult child had been harder than any other experience in their lives. They realized that they had an inner strength previously unknown. The words of a 58-year-old grandmother who began raising three grandchildren after her daughter died from a drug overdose describes some of the strength she discovered,

> My daughter was staying with this guy, who was on paint, and with his parents who both drank. Well I kept saying, "I can't keep helping you" but in my heart I knew I would. His mother called me in the middle of the night she said "Come over here and get your daughter before he kills her," so I go over there. She said "Well he's kicked me in the stomach" and I said "Well he won't do it while I'm here–get your stuff and put it in my car and I'm taking you home with me." Well he kicked her again, and I went in there right in the middle of it, and I said "You do that again boy, and I'm gonna kill you right here, you lay a hand on her again and I'm gonna kill you," and I heard these feet hit the floor and I knew it was his dad and I thought oh my God I'm gonna have to fight the two of them, here come his dad in there he said "No you're not, because if he does it again I'll kill him myself." You know there was reason for me to have to go through this. Let me tell you something I never used to have that strength–I used to just cry.

A 62-year-old grandmother who is raising a 14-year-old granddaughter also illustrates,

> When my daughter's husband beat her up and, dragged her out in the front yard he grabbed my granddaughter, Rebecca, and told her that she'd never see her mother again. After she'd been through this it was kind of touch and go. That was the worst, absolute positive worst time. It was terrifying. I never knew that I could be so persistent about anything but you just do it because it is yours to do. Looking back on it, I wonder sometimes how I had the nerve do some of the things I did. But when you are worried about your child and your grandchild, you can do a lot of things you might not do otherwise. I never gave a lot of thought to what I had to do, other than doing it, it's all a necessity. Because I've always been kind of mild mannered but if you've got someone you love threatened,

you'd be surprised what you'd do to defend them and make sure they're ok. We had to take the Emergency Protective Order to her pre-school; we had to take it to public school when she went to public school. It showed that he couldn't come to school and get her. It was awful, it was just awful. And, my daughter was beside herself and I was beside myself worried about what he was going to do next.

The experiences of grandmothers who are raising grandchildren change the caregivers in many ways. The discovery of internal strength was important recognition for women who had previously seen themselves as powerless.

DISCUSSION

Events that trigger the need for grandparent caregiving cause dramatic changes in the relationship between an older adult and her grandchild. A grandmother's home may provide temporary shelter for a child during troubled times when a parent's behavior is erratic, or it may become permanent if a parent is unable to gain control of the disruptive problems. Knowledge about the special needs of grandparent caregivers is important because the sometimes-transient nature of grandparent caregiving may mean that society is aware of only the tip of the iceberg. This special type of family caregiving bears both important similarities and differences to other types of family caregiving.

Family relationships are of primary importance to the grandmother caregivers in this study, who expressed intense and ongoing worry about their adult child even if contact had been completely severed. Women who fill this caregiving role in multigenerational families concern themselves with the well being of their adult child and their grandchild(ren) simultaneously. This same issue is similarly reflected nationwide. Previous studies have found that two-thirds of all grandparent caregivers are the linking generation who may be doing "double duty" in simultaneously caring for both a grandchild and an impaired adult child (Burnette, 1999c; Fuller-Thompson, Minkler, & Driver, 1997). Despite difficult and sometimes tragic problems, grandmother caregivers continue to hope for positive changes in their adult child's life, and to work for the well being of all generations in their families.

The balance of work and family responsibilities added a new type of strain for some of the grandmother caregivers who participated in this study. Many grandmother caregivers returned to work, or arranged work at home to help offset the additional financial burden of caring for their grandchildren later in life. Health insurance for grandchildren, child care and missed work time are new issues for women who had not worked outside the home while their children were young. Issues of health insurance coverage for grandchildren are complicated by a skipped generation of parental authority. Grandmother caregivers also found additional support and understanding among friends and colleagues on their jobs.

The emotional repercussions from a family crisis of this magnitude are notable for both grandparents and grandchildren. Grandmothers who are raising grandchildren may be dealing with conflicting feelings about their adult child and grandchild. Grandchildren may have been victims of prolonged physical or verbal abuse, and they may also have been neglected. Emotional responses to grandparent caregiving may include many simultaneous complex feelings such as guilt, anger at an adult child, and grief from multiple serious losses (Burnette, 1999b; Minkler & Roe, 1993). Grandchildren's behaviors may reflect their traumatic experiences in a dysfunctional home situation (Shore & Hayslip, 1994). Intense emotions accompany all types of family caregiving, but both the source and outcomes are different when caregiving follows a family upheaval, which necessitates grandparent caregiving.

The stress of raising a grandchild has effects on caregivers' mental and physical health. Grandmother caregivers in this study expressed feeling fatigue and a need to talk about their feelings. Grandmother caregivers may deny their own health problems as a way of coping with extra burden and instead, focus all their attention on the needs of a grandchild (Minkler & Roe, 1993). Healthcare professionals who work with multigenerational families need to be aware of the potential coexistence of health and mental health problems in both children and their grandparent caregivers. Caregivers who experience mental and emotional strain have a higher chance of mortality than those who do not (Shulz & Beach, 1999).

Complex multi-problem situations exist in many grandparent-headed families. A sense of social isolation and exhaustion can stem from the new responsibilities and uncertainties that accompany grandparent caregiving. Feelings of changed or lost identity may result from becoming engulfed in the caregiver role (Pearlin, Mullan, Semple, & Skaff, 1990). The advent of grandparent caregiving replaces some of the simple joys of grandparent-grandchild relationships with new challenges. Grandmother caregivers described discovering internal strength during intense times of conflict or fear. Grandmother caregivers' lives are changed by the challenges of raising their childrens' children. Caregivers' reflections about the experience highlight important meaning they find in caring for the youngest most vulnerable members of society.

Implications for Practice

The organization entitled "Strengthening Aging and Gerontology Education for Social Work" declares that family caregiving is an intergenerational issue that permeates many areas of social work practice. Family caregivers cite social workers as an important source of information and education (National Alliance for Caregiving, 1997), and caregiver support is seen as a vital social work role. Stress, caregiver burden, and the mental health needs of caregivers are not adequately addressed by the medical profession and are a natural area of service or social workers (SAGE-SW, 1999). Recognition of the special and unique issues faced by grandmother caregivers is important for social workers, who may interact with all generations of families in a variety of settings.

Awareness about the similarities and differences among diverse groups of caregivers is an important future issue for the social work profession. Knowledge of the unique and special needs of different types of family caregivers can promote more effective social work advocacy for groups who have previously been marginalized. Caregiving is a life span issue with many applications for social work curriculum (SAGE-SW, 1999). Social workers may encounter family caregivers in a variety of agency settings, including those primarily focused on children and adolescents. Both the burdens and benefits of providing care for a dependent loved one are important considerations in successful work with a family system. Future research with family caregivers will provide important additional insight for the social work profession.

REFERENCES

Auslander, G., & Litwin, H. (1990). Social support networks and formal help seeking: Differences between applicants to social services and a non-applicant sample. *Journals of Gerontolgy: Social Sciences, 45*, S112-119.

Barer, B., & Johnson, C. L. (1990). A critique of the caregiving literature. *The Gerontologist, 30(1),* 26-29.

Baum, M., & Page, M. (1991). Caregiving and multigenerational families. *The Gerontologist, 31(6),* 762-769.

Biegel, D. E., & Shulz, R. (1999). Caregiving and caregiver interventions in aging and mental illness. *Family Relations, 48(4),* 345-360.

Bowers, B. F., & Myers, B. J. (1999). Grandmothers providing care for grandchildren: Consequences of various levels of caregiving. *Family Relations, 14(3)*, 330-311.

Brody, E. M. (1981). Women in the middle and family help to older people. *The Gerontologist, 21*(5), 471-480.

Burnette, D. (1999a). Custodial grandparents in Latino families: Patterns of service use and predictors of unmet needs. *Social Work, 44(*1), 22-27.

Burnette, D. (1999). Physical and emotional well being of custodial grandparents in Latino families. *American Journal of Orthopsychiatry, 69*(3), 305-309.

Burnette, D. (1999). Social relationships of Latino grandparent caregivers: A role theory perspective. *The Gerontologist, 39*(1), 49-56.

Burton, L. M. (1992). Black grandparents rearing children of drug-addicted parents: Stressors, outcomes, and social service needs. *The Gerontologist, 32*, 744-751.

Fuller-Thomson, E., Minkler, M., & Driver, D. (1997). A profile of grandparents raising grandchildren in the United States. *The Gerontologist, 37*(3), 406-411.

Joslin, D., & Brouard, A. (1995). The prevalence of grandmothers as primary caregivers in a poor pediatric population. *Journal of Community Health, 20*, 383-401.

Kaufman, A. V. (1998). Older parents who care for adult children with serious mental illness. *The Journal of Gerontological Social Work, 29*(4), 35-53.

Kramer, B. J. (1997). Gain in the caregiving experience: Where are we? What next? *The Gerontologist, 37*(2), 218-232.

Kramer B. J., & Kipnis, S. (1995). Eldercare and work-role conflict: Toward an understanding of gender differences in caregiver burden. *The Gerontologist, 35*(3), 340-348.

Lefley, H. P. (1996). Aging parents as caregivers of mentally ill adult children: An emerging social problem. *Hospital and Community Psychiatry, 38*, 1063-1063.

Lugaila, T. (1998). Marital status and living arrangements: March 1997 (Current Population Report Series, P20-506). Suitland, MD: U.S. Bureau of the Census.

McRae, H. (1998). Managing feelings: Caregiving as emotion work. *Research on Aging, 20*(1), 137-160.

Minkler, M. (1999). Intergenerational households headed by grandparents: Contexts, realities, and implications for policy. *Journal of Aging Studies, 13*(2), 199-209.

Minkler, M., & Roe, K. M. (1993). *Grandmothers as caregivers: Raising children of the crack cocaine epidemic.* Newbury Park: Sage.

Moen, P., & Dempster-McClain, D. (1989). Social integration and longevity: An event history analysis of women's roles and resilience. *American Sociological Review, 54*(August), 635-647.

National Alliance for Caregiving. (1997). Family caregiving in the U.S.: Findings from a national survey. www.http://caregiving.org/.

Pearlin, L. I., Mullan, J. T., Semple, S. J., & Skaf, M. M. (1990). Caregiving and the stress process: An overview of concepts and their measures. *The Gerontologist, 30*(5), 583-591.

Penrod, J. D., Kane, R. A., Kane, R. L., & Finch, M. D. (1995). Who cares? The size, scope, and composition of the caregiver support system. *The Gerontologist, 35*(4), 489-497.

Pruchno, R. (1999). Raising grandchildren: The experiences of black and white grandmothers. *The Gerontologist, 39*(2), 209-221.

Pruchno, R. A., Burant, C. J., & Peters, N. D. (1997). Typologies of caregiving families: Family congruence and individual well-being. *The Gerontologist, 37*(2), 157-167.

Roe, K. M., & Minkler, M. (1998). Grandparents raising grandchildren: Challenges and responses. *Generations, 22*(4), 25-32.

Roe, K. M., Minkler, M., Saunders, F., & Thomson, G. E. (1996). Health of grandmothers raising children of the crack cocaine epidemic. *Medical Care, 34*, 1072-1084.

Ryff, C. D. (1989). Happiness is everything, or is it? Explorations on the meaning of psychological well-being. *Journal of Personality and Social Psychology, 57*, 1069-1081.

SAGE-SW. (1999, Fall). Strengthening Aging and Gerontology Education for Social Work Newsletter. New York: CSWE.

Sands, R. G., & Goldberg-Glen, R. S. (1998). The impact of employment and serious illness on grandmothers who are raising their grandchildren. *Journal of Women and Aging, 10*(3), 41-58.

Sharlach, A. E. (1994). Caregiving and employment: Competing or complementary roles? *The Gerontologist, 34*(3), 378-385.

Shore, R. J., & Hayslip, B. (1994). Custodial grandparenting: Implications for children's development. In A. E. Gottfried & A. W. Gottfried (Eds.), *Redefining families: Implications for children's development* (pp. 171-217). New York: Plenum Press.

Shulz, R., & Beach, S. R. (1999). Caregiving as a risk factor for mortality: The caregiver health study. *JAMA, December 15.*

Skaff, M. M., & Pearlin, L. I. (1992). Caregiving: Role engulfment and loss of self. *The Gerontologist, 32*(5), 656-664.

Strawbridge, W. J., Wallhagen, M. I., Shema, S. J., & Kaplan, G. A. (1997). New burdens or more of the same? Comparing grandparent, spouse, and adult-child caregivers. The *Gerontologist, 37*(4), 505-510.

Thiede-Call, K., Finch, M. A., Huck, S. M., & Kane, R. A. (1999). Caregiver burden from a social exchange perspective: Caring for older people after hospital discharge. *Journal of Marriage and the Family, 61*(3), 688-699.

Zarit, S. H., Reever, K. E., & Bach-Peterson, J. (1980). Relatives of the impaired elderly: Correlates of feelings of burden. *The Gerontologist, 20*(6), 649-655.

Empowerment Theory
and Long-Living Women:
A Feminist and Disability Perspective

Carolyn Morell

SUMMARY. Empowerment theory is central to social work and to feminist gerontology. Yet an emphasis on increasing power and control over the circumstances of one's life does not neatly "fit" the involuntary bodily realities that figure centrally in the experiences of late age. The project of this article is to argue that the paradox of late life empowerment is that it requires acceptance and affirmation of the weak, suffering, and uncontrollable body. *[Article copies available for a fee from The Haworth Document Delivery Service: 1-800-HAWORTH. E-mail address: <docdelivery@ haworthpress.com> Website: <http://www.HaworthPress.com> © 2003 by The Haworth Press, Inc. All rights reserved.]*

KEYWORDS. Feminism, empowerment, gerontology, women, disability

Those who are weak have great difficulty finding their place in our society. The image of the ideal human as powerful and capable disenfranchises the old, the sick, the less-abled . . .

(Vanier, 1998, p. 45)

Carolyn Morell, PhD, is affiliated with the Social Work Department, P.O. #1942, Niagara University, Niagara, NY 14109 (E-mail: morellc@niagara.edu).

[Haworth co-indexing entry note]: "Empowerment Theory and Long-Living Women: A Feminist and Disability Perspective." Morell, Carolyn. Co-published simultaneously in *Journal of Human Behavior in the Social Environment* (The Haworth Social Work Practice Press, an imprint of The Haworth Press, Inc.) Vol. 7, No. 3/4, 2003, pp. 225-236; and: *Women and Girls in the Social Environment: Behavioral Perspectives* (ed: Nancy J. Smyth) The Haworth Social Work Practice Press, an imprint of The Haworth Press, Inc., 2003, pp. 225-236. Single or multiple copies of this article are available for a fee from The Haworth Document Delivery Service [1-800-HAWORTH, 9:00 a.m. - 5:00 p.m. (EST). E-mail address: docdelivery@haworthpress.com].

http://www.haworthpress.com/store/product.asp?sku=J137
© 2003 by The Haworth Press, Inc. All rights reserved.
Digital Object Identifier: 10.1300/J137v7n03_13

Empowerment theory is central to social work and to feminist gerontology (Garner, 1999). For social workers, empowerment involves emphasizing strengths and capacities and increasing personal, interpersonal, and political power through engaged energetic action (Browne, 1998; Gutierrez, 1990; Simon, 1994). This conceptualization of empowerment is helpful with many client groups, but when considering the experiences of long-living women, empowerment theory seems somehow inadequate and age-biased. Privileging power and seeking control over the circumstances of one's life does not neatly "fit" the involuntary bodily realities that figure centrally in experiences of late age. With advanced age, the limits of human existence come into sharp focus and pose challenges to our profession's ideas about empowerment.

The project of this article is to argue that age-sensitive empowerment theory must become "embodied," and in doing so, accept human powerlessness and embrace human weakness. To begin, I briefly consider the contemporary landscape of long life and contend that late life is a "women's issue" and a "disability issue." Then, in order to explore the meaning of empowerment for women in their late years, I draw on the insights of feminist disability theorists as well as historians and ethicists. I end up arguing that the paradox of late life empowerment is that it requires us to affirm the weak, suffering, and uncontrollable body.[1]

LATE LIFE AS A "WOMEN'S ISSUE" AND A "DISABILITY ISSUE"

The demographics of an aging population call out for innovative theorizing about women and late life empowerment. The fastest growing population category in Western countries is people age eighty-five and older, and women are the clear majority of this group. Women continue to outlive men and are therefore more likely than men to experience whatever advanced age brings. One set of well-documented age correlates is a multitude of chronic illnesses, diseases and disabilities. For instance, by the age of eighty-five, fifty percent of women will need assistance with daily living, and by the age of seventy-five, most women will have at least one, and on average two, chronic conditions or disabilities (Callahan, 1999). Not surprisingly, a demographic profile of Americans who are one hundred years old and over reveals that nearly eighty percent are women, and nearly fifty percent of those women live in nursing homes. While many centenarians are relatively healthy and mobile, over half see long life as a burden because of physical and/or mental disabilities (Ramirez, 1999). Of course no centenarian has the physical vitality s/he had fifty years earlier.

Long-living women have to confront problematic changes in the body that accompany long life and also the stigmas related to these changes in appearance and functioning. These negative marks rooted in age and gender are manifested in a wide range of phenomena, both on individual and institutional levels–stereotypes and myths, ridicule, dislike, and avoidance (Butler, 1975), and discriminatory policies in housing, employment and all manner of services. Both men and women are oppressed by ageism, yet women experience additional insults related to the double standard of aging and their greater economic vulnerability compared to men. The combined negative impact of age, gender (and for many women race and/or ethnicity), and economic location leads Pearsall (1997) to assert that long-living women in Western countries experience the most stigmatized location in the life course. These stigmas relate directly to the aged body.

Aging is an embodied phenomenon, yet social workers have not fully included the body in our empowerment discourse. Medical perspectives make the body central, but they apply a model of youth and health and thus disempower elders by defining the aging body as evidence of biological failure and inferiority. We need to theorize embodiment in a way that provides an alternative, liberating meaning. Scholars from a variety of disciplines, who understand the body as a site of oppression and empowerment, can help social workers build a theory of late life empowerment.

In the following pages, a summary of some exciting theoretical work that has been done recently by feminist philosophers and disability theorists, historians, and ethicists is presented. With their insights, I argue that the myth of bodily control is especially oppressive for women who live into late age. I maintain that late life empowerment must forefront accommodation of the old and disabled body, and thus empowering long-living women involves validating the whole of the human condition, which includes experiences of weakness and powerlessness.

OPPRESSION AND THE MYTH OF BODILY CONTROL

Susan Wendell is a feminist philosopher and disability theorist whose work has useful applications for late life empowerment. While her focus is primarily on disability and not age (although her most recent article *is* about old women), her insights apply to women who are living late life (many of whom are or will be disabled). Below I present key aspects of her perspective on disability and relate it to the situations of long-living women.

In her book titled, *The Rejected Body: Feminist Philosophical Reflections on Disability* (1996), Wendell describes how in North America the idealization of the body as young and healthy leads directly to the marginalization of people who are disabled and old. Implied in any body idealization is the rejection of some kinds of bodies and some facets of bodily life. She uses the term "the rejected body" to refer to bodily experiences that are "feared, ignored, despised, and/or rejected in a society and its culture" (p. 85). Illness, disability, weakness, bodily suffering and death, as well as deviations from the cultural ideals of bodily appearance constitute "the rejected body."

Contemplation of change and loss is often frightening. Most people who grow up in Western cultures fear loss of bodily control. Unfortunately, this fear leads to denial and flight from confrontation with the rejected and devalued body. Individuals experience both cultural and internal pressures to deny bodily weakness and to dread old age. We may feel ashamed about our distance from cultural ideals of the body. Yet long-living women must struggle harder than younger women for an identity that is both positive and realistic. Said simply, long-living women are measured by an impossible standard–a healthy youthful "feminine" body. And when women cannot measure up, they become devalued as people because of their devalued bodies (Hannaford, 1985). When long-living women internalize these values, they may experience self-alienation.

A major barrier to accepting the full reality of bodily life in all its variability is "the widespread myth that the body can be controlled" (Wendell, 1996, p. 93). The main idea of the myth of control is that human beings can prevent illness, disability, and death by means of self-control and appropriate choices. The celebrated notion of "successful aging" can be used to illustrate the oppressive nature of the myth of control.

The ideal of "successful aging" has gained popularity in the past two decades. This goal is promoted vigorously by a market economy, by many doctors and undoubtedly by some social workers (indeed I have been guilty of promoting this ideal). Through the exercise of self-control, so the story goes, women who eat properly, become physically fit, think positively, reduce stress, consume the right mix of vitamins and minerals, and replace their hormones can stay healthy and youthful. We can age "successfully," meaning we can eliminate or postpone the aging process. An older woman who does not fit the active, healthy youthful image is unsuccessful at aging, a failure–even if she is successfully living with a variety of challenging physical problems or disabilities.

This myth of control, with its rejection of actual lived experience, serves women poorly. Combined with the dominant image of the acceptable body, the control myth is clearly disempowering. Women are pressured to control their bodies (an impossible task) in order to create an acceptable body (an impossible goal). Wendell (1999) in her most recent publication about late life women titled, "Old Women Out of Control," articulates the oppressive nature of insisting on the ideal of a wonderful and successful aging:

> . . . leaning on a distinction between normal and sick/disabled middle and old age is no solution to the problem of being excluded by age from identifying oneself, and being identified by others, as having a valuable present and future life. It benefits some–those who are aging in good health with little or no disability–at the expense of others, *including their probable future selves*, on whom the demeaning narratives of decline can and will be projected. (p. 134)

Representing late life as a splendid time in which we can empower ourselves through the use of willpower and proper actions does not reflect the full reality. "Aging is not always and never *just* being sick and dying, but it is also these" (Wendell, 1999, pp. 134-135).

Of course healthy practices are appropriate and life-style choices make a difference. For example, those who don't smoke live longer, and better, lives. Yet we are offered ideologies of self-control that "allow us to hope to avoid the unsuccessful version of late life at a price; we are blamed (and may blame ourselves) should we become sick or disabled" (Wendell, 1999, p. 137).

Wendell (1996) points out that feminist theorists have successfully critiqued the oppressive impact of the idealization of women's bodies but have promoted our own body ideals that reinforce the myth of control and exclude disabled (and long-living) women:

> We have celebrated those aspects of women's bodily experience that are sources of pleasure, satisfaction, and feelings of connection, but we have underestimated the bodily frustration and suffering that social justice cannot prevent or relieve. Feminists have criticized and worked to undo men's control of women's bodies

without undermining the myth that women can control our own
bodies. (pp. 92-93)

Wendell calls on feminists to confront the weak, suffering and uncontrollable body in theorizing and in practice, since the myth of control is
a major contributor to the stigmas surrounding old age and disability.

Disability theorists are not the only scholars who have identified the
myth of control as an oppressive force in the life of elders and people
with disabilities. In *The Journey of Life: A Cultural History of Aging in
America* (1997), Thomas Cole describes the rise of the burdensome
myth of control (without calling it this) in North America during the
mid-1800s. Before this time, old age embodiment was not stigmatized
and feared but was acceptable, even honorable. Most women and men
lived in families and communities regulated by social and religious
principles and existentially nourishing views of aging predominated
(Cole, 1997). The realities of physical decline and death were infused
with meaning as people brought themselves into alignment with the
eternal order of the universe. Aging was primarily viewed as an issue
requiring moral and spiritual commitment. In short, before the middle
of the nineteenth century, the "intractable sorrows and infirmities of age
remained culturally acceptable" (p. 230). Growing old had a positive
meaning and significance for the individual and the community. The
end of life was seen as a time of paradoxes, a place of wisdom and suffering, spiritual growth and physical decline, honor and vulnerability.

With the dawn of the Victorian era, attitudes toward aging changed
along with the culture. The majority of North Americans began to view
aging "not as a fated aspect of individual and social existence but as one
of life's problems to be solved through willpower, aided by science,
technology, and expertise" (Cole, 1997, p. xxii). In the Victorian era, a
rigid polarity of positive and negative stereotypes about aging replaced
the dignified views of earlier times. The growth of liberal individualism
gave rise to a moral code requiring physical self-control to master old
age, and elders were morally pressured to age well. People who worked
hard and disciplined themselves could preserve health and independence; those who were lazy and undisciplined were doomed to a misera-
ble old age (Cole, 1997, p. xxvi).

After World War II, the meaning of aging again changed with a
changing culture. With the ascendency of medicine and science, aging
became medicalized. Today's goal of the scientific management of aging–the maximization of health and organic functioning–is a goal that
generally ignores human limits and eclipses the existential dimensions

of aging and "overlooks the spiritual resources needed to redeem human finitude" (Cole, 1997, p. xxv).

Hope for full control of the body is fueled by the fact that more control is possible today than ever before. New drugs, surgeries, and social programs allow levels of control never before imagined. The novelist Fay Weldon (2000) writes, at age 67, that "by now I'd have been dead once if it weren't for antibiotics and twice if not for surgery" (p. 2).

But these significant changes in length and quality of life do not mean that we control life. And it is the myth that we *can* control bodily life that dominates cultural discussions of aging today. Advances in genetic and cellular technologies turn into promises of the fountain of youth. Even death is considered to be conquerable. The scientific managers of aging encourage us to think about growing old not as part of the human condition but as a problem to be controlled and solved. Then when our bodies do go out of control, we feel a deep sense of shame and others are revolted. The feelings of shame and revulsion reflect our society's continuing and apparently intractable hostility to physical decline and mental decay which is imposed "with particular vengeance on older women" (Cole, 1997, p. xxiv).

Cole (1997) summarizes the dilemma and the problem with our scientific control of aging well: " . . . no amount of biomedical research and technical intervention can bring aging fully under the control of human will or desire. Growing old and dying, like being born and growing up, will remain part of the cycle of organic life, part of the coming into being and passing away that make up the history of the universe" (Cole, 1997, p. xxv).

EMPOWERMENT:
ACCOMMODATION AND AFFIRMATION
OF THE UNCONTROLLABLE BODY

The myth of bodily control is a privatizing and thus personal model of disability which undermines social responsibility for an aging (and disabled) population. In contrast, feminist disability and historical perspectives are roped to the social world and focus on hostile social arrangements, not on controlling bodies and minds that are judged inferior. A social model of disability is well articulated in the 1990 Americans With Disabilities Act:

> . . . the 1990 Americans With Disabilities Act is thoroughly grounded in the belief that disability is socially constructed . . . Be-

cause it attributes the dysfunctions of individuals with physical, sensory, and cognitive impairments mainly to their being situated in hostilely built and organized environments, the social model of disability construes the isolation of people with disabilities (and by implication of elderly people as well) as the correctable product of how such individuals interact with stigmatizing social values and debilitating social arrangements rather than as the unavoidable outcome of their impairments. (Silvers, 1999, pp. 214-15)

Clearly the United States is not prepared for the large numbers of women who will need accommodation in the future, given disabilities connected to longevity. Planning to accommodate age-related disabilities is in the best interests of everyone. Yet such planning is hampered because those who make policy and the general public "prefer to imagine that they will age and die without experiencing disability" (Wendell, 1999, p. 135).

Because we believe the body can be controlled, much of the world is structured as if everyone were "physically strong . . . as though everyone can walk, see and hear well, as though everyone can work and play at a pace that is not compatible with any kind of illness or pain, as though no one is ever dizzy or incontinent or simply needs to sit or lie down" (Wendell, 1989, p. 69). Architecture as well as most of the physical and social organization of life assumes that we are either healthy and strong and able-bodied or that we are completely disabled, unable to participate in life. The public world is made for the strong and able-bodied. The private world is the world of the rejected body. Long-living people and people with disabilities lose out on important social options and opportunities, while people who are temporarily young and without physical limitations remain in the grips of the myth that the body can be controlled, that disability and perhaps even death, can be prevented.

Oppression related to the myth of control is not one of environmental neglect alone but of the negative meanings assigned to old age. Silvers (1999) reminds us that neither growing years nor decreasing competence drives the social process that relegates elders to meaningless roles since young, capable individuals are also subject to role devaluation if their bodies become disabled. Elders and younger people with disabilities experience marginalization because their physical and cognitive styles of performance differ from those of the socially dominant group, namely, younger males (Silvers, 1999). Cast as an inferior class, elders and those with physical, sensory, or cognitive impairments are isolated and given a roleless role and placed on the margins of community life.

Writing of people with disabilities, Harlan Hahn (1987) makes the point that "the pervasive sense of physical and social isolation" experienced by people with disabilities is produced by restrictions of the built environment and also by the aversive reactions of the non-disabled. This holds true for elders as well. Assignment to a meaningless existence (apart from "successfully aging" which fails as bodies fail) is an arrangement that social workers and other social scientists "warn against perpetuating because the individuals assigned to them are highly exposed to psychosocial risk" (Silvers, 1999, p. 211).

Replenishing the cultural meanings of late life involves thinking about bodily difference as diversity rather than deviancy. Disability theorist and activist Carol J. Gill's (1994) thoughts about the ideal world for people with disabilities are applicable to long-living women. I adopt Gill's vision and apply it to elder women in the following paragraph.

In the ideal world, old women's body-based differentness from younger others would not be devalued, but accepted as part of human diversity. There would be respectful curiosity about what women have learned from the process of growing old that could be contributed to others. In such a world, women would not mind being called "old." "Being unable to do something the way most people do it would not be seen as something bad that needed curing. It would be seen as just a difference" (Gill, 1994, p. 45). Differences might make old women proficient in some contexts, deficient in others, or not matter at all. For example, if a long-living woman can't run, she might be an inferior messenger if time is a critical factor. However, her inability to run might just stimulate her to address time more creatively or to develop ways to send messages swiftly that are as efficient as running, or vastly superior. In other words, even if she had a difference that might hinder her in some contexts, she wouldn't be judged *generally* deficient because a recognized feature of an age-accepting culture would be the fact that such limitations may be related to innovation and inventiveness.

We can also turn to spiritual traditions for a source of renewed meaning for old age. While certain problems of aging may be alleviated, other problems, such as the gradual decline of energy and vitality and the eventual path to death, are intractable. Our culture's ability to infuse these existential realities with vital meaning has profoundly deteriorated over the past two centuries. The medical model of aging has obliterated the existential dimension of aging. Yet, as we enter the twenty-first century, there is growing interest in the development of satisfying spiritual and cosmic views on aging (Cole, 1997).

Philosopher and ethicist Margaret Urban Walker (1999) describes how many cultures have understood late life as a time that is ripe for spiritual work, for contemplation, for counseling and guiding others. She asserts that there is no reason for us to cease *living* a valuable life in very late years with old and frail bodies. With awareness, capacities for feeling and opportunities to belong to or with something larger than oneself, the existential meanings of life's later times can be recovered. Feminist disability theorists such as Susan Wendell (1989; 1996; 1999), Barbara Hillyer (1993; 1998), and Nancy Mairs (1996) advocate acknowledgment of how disability can stimulate mental, emotional, moral, and spiritual growth and cultivation of "the demanding arts of acceptance, adjustment, and appreciation" (Wendell, 1999, p. 146).

Said simply, the empowerment of long-living women from age oppression involves environmental and ideological change. The out-of-control body needs to be accommodated, and nourishing meanings of late life need to be cultivated. With these changes, the aged body will no longer be feared, ignored, despised, and rejected. Interventions at the social level and the symbolic level can dignify aging once again and make growing old socially acceptable.

CONCLUSION

As social workers committed to late life empowerment, we must struggle against a strict medical model which emphasizes embodiment to the exclusion of empowerment. Yet we must struggle against an empowerment model that emphasizes power to the exclusion of embodiment as well. I believe that in social work theory and practice we must temper our eager promotion of strengths, competence, and energy that inadvertently reinforces the myth of bodily control and risks rejection of the less-than-energetic, less-than-competent body. We must work to empower powerlessness.

As social workers we want to assist people in exercising power in their lives. Equally important and often neglected is encouraging people of all ages to acknowledge that "human beings are limited; that some losses cannot be repaired; and above all that strength and weakness must be integrated" (Hillyer, 1993, p. 15). An age-aware and body-sensitive model of empowerment recognizes that we are powerful and we are powerless.

Empowerment theory, in its confrontation with oppression, requires recognition of our *full* human condition.

NOTE

1. I intentionally use a subjective voice throughout this article. One of the distinctive features of feminist inquiry is insistence that the author appear as a real, historical individual with specifically stated interests and desires rather than an invisible and objective voice of authority. In this article, my goal is to present a compelling argument with the hope of stimulating thoughtful dialogue on a subject of collective concern.

REFERENCES

Browne, C. V. (1998). *Women, feminism, and aging.* New York: Springer.
Butler, R. N. (1975). *Why Survive?* New York: Harper & Row.
Callahan, D. (1999). Age, sex, and resource allocation. In *Mother time: Women, aging and ethics,* Margaret Urban Walker. New York: Rowman & Littlefield Publishers, Inc.
Cole, T. R. (1997). *The journey of life: A cultural history of aging in America.* New York: Cambridge University Press, Canto edition.
Garner, J. D. (1999). Feminism and feminist gerontology. In *Fundamentals of feminist gerontology,* ed. J. Dianne Garner. New York: The Haworth Press, Inc.
Gill, C. J. (1994). Questioning continuum. In *The ragged edge: The disability experience from the pages of the first fifteen years of the disability rag,* ed. Barrett Shaw. Louisville, KY: The Advocado Press.
Gutierrez, L. M. (1990). Working with women of color: An empowerment perspective. In *Social Work* 35 (2): 179-192.
Hahn, H. (1987). Civil rights for disabled americans. In *Images of the disabled, disabling images,* ed. Alan Gartner and Tome Joe. New York: Praeger.
Hannaford, S. (1985). *Living outside inside. A disabled woman's experience. Towards a social and political perspective.* Berkeley: Canterbury Press.
Hillyer, B. (1993). *Feminism and disability.* Norman: University of Oklahoma Press.
Hillyer, B. (1998). Embodiment of older women: Silences. In *Frontiers: A journal of women's studies,* 19 (1): 48-60.
Mairs, N. (1996). *Waist-high in the world: A life among the nondisabled.* Boston: Beacon Press.
Pearsall, M. (1997). *The other within us: Feminist explorations of women and aging.* Boulder: Westview Press.
Ramirez, L. (1999). "Fastest-growing segment in U.S. is centenarians." *The Buffalo Evening News,* August 18, p. A8.
Silvers, A. (1999). Aging fairly: Feminist and disability perspectives on intergenerational justice. In *Mother time: Women, aging, and ethics,* ed. Margaret Urban Walker. New York: Rowman & Littlefield Publishers, Inc.

Simon, B. L. (1994). *The empowerment tradition in american social work: A history.* New York: Columbia University Press.

Vanier, J. (1998). *Becoming human.* Toronto: House of Anansi Press Limited.

Walker, M. U. (1999). Getting out of line: Alternatives to life as a career. In *Mother time: Women, aging, and ethics,* ed. Margaret Urban Walker. New York: Rowman & Littlefield Publishers, Inc.

Weldon, F. (2000). The rise of the ergonarchy. In *New Statesmen,* April 17. http://www.consider.net/forum, 1-8.

Wendell, S. (1989). Toward a feminist theory of disability. In *Hypatia,* 4 (2): 63-81.

Wendell, S. (1996). *The rejected body: Feminist philosophical reflections on disability.* New York: Routledge.

Wendell, S. (1999). Old women out of control: Some thoughts on aging, ethics, and psychosomatic medicine. In *Mother time: Women, aging, and ethics,* ed. Margaret Urban Walker. New York: Rowman & Littlefield Publishers, Inc.

Index